A LINE IN THE SAND

Jim Coons

All scripture quoted is from Today's New International Version unless otherwise noted.

Dedication

This book is dedicated to Emily, Julia, Jakob, and Eliza Kate—my beautiful family. "When you undergo treatments and surgeries," Julia wisely once said, "we all do undergo treatments and surgeries." We have battled cancer these past several years, each in our unique way. You are the reason I fight so hard and allow them to cut and chemo me. I want to grow old with you, walk you down the aisles, hold your children, and raise you as people of deep faith, a huge capacity to love and be loved, integrity, and hope that this life is not all there is. There is more!

Contents

Acknowledgments

I would like to thank my *Army of Love*, the community of love and support that surrounds me, because you thought my *CarePage* entries should be published in a book form. I had my doubts that I could do it and some difficult moments reading back through some of the most intense moments of my life. It was hard, but it was good. This amazing community pushed and reminded me week after that my words were helping them and their friends. I am grateful that my journey is bringing good in this world. I am humbled.

I especially want to thank Lisa Christiansen and Nora Profit for putting legs on my dream to write. You each helped me believe in my ability to share my story in words. A huge debt of gratitude goes out to Katherine Hilzer for editing my jumbled thoughts.

I cannot imagine these last few years without my family and close friends. For those I have called at 2 A.M. and have talked me off multiple ledges, thank you. You make life worth fighting for!

I also pay my deep respect to my oncologist, Dr. Sam Mazj and the myriad of oncology nurses and staff who have administered not just chemo and healing medicines, but hope. They are God's instruments of healing!

Finally, I thank God for the passion and ability to write. It is to him that I pray these words fall on fertile soil.

"There's nothing like a brush with mortality to put things into perspective. Everything comes into sharper focus, you really appreciate what you might have lost. If you think you may not be able to sing again, well, then you're not going to mess around."

-BONO

U2 by U2

Introduction

I love Line Drawers. Line Drawers are gutsy, stubborn, picky people who refuse to be defined by their circumstances. They have discovered their limits, and when the walls of life close in around them they know when to reach down and draw a line in the sand. They draw a line in the sand between themselves and their circumstances and say, "Enough is enough! No more! You don't have permission to cross this line!" They have the rare ability to filter through the voices telling them who they ought to be, what they ought to think, and how they ought to believe. They don't buy it. They are people of conviction and know who they are, what they think, and what they believe and live accordingly. They are fierce individuals who have learned the art of tuning their ears, minds, and hearts to a higher Voice that reminds them of a deeper truth: Their identities are not their circumstances.

I have stage three colon cancer and every day as I wake up I am faced with the decision about who I will be: Jim Coons the cancer patient, or just Jim. Some days I give in and play the role of the patient. I sit around feeling sorry for myself whining, "Why me? What did I do to deserve this?" I allow others to feel sorry for me and treat me like a helpless child. I feel sick and depressed because I have cancer and lack the energy to be a husband, dad, pastor or friend. I may as well get measured for my coffin on those days.

But on better days I wake up with clenched teeth, a clear mind, and ready to send cancer back to hell where it came from. I don't feel sorry for myself on these days, but remember that before I had cancer, I was just Jim. I hear the higher Voice, God's voice, reminding me that apart from cancer clinics, hospitals, blood tests, PET scans, surgeries, and chemotherapy, I am just Jim: A son, brother, husband, dad, fly-fisherman, music lover, book reader, cyclist, pastor, and Child of the Living God. Cancer can't rob me of these deep truths—I won't let it. This is my line in the sand.

Since being diagnosed with cancer three years ago, I have been inspired by people who are Line Drawers. They have helped me determine when and where to draw my own lines. Jesus of Nazareth was the original Line Drawer. Talk about a stubborn person! He refused time and again to allow others to define him, regardless of their expectations. He drew a line between himself and Satan in the desert at the beginning of his public ministry (Luke 4:1-13). He wouldn't let the devil compromise his identity, his power or his role as Savior. Again, he drew a line between himself and the expectations of others when he denied being a prophet to Peter and the other disciples (Mark 8:27-30). And he drew a line between himself and death when he rolled away the gravestone and rose from the dead (John 20). The guy drew some serious lines! And he taught others how to draw their lines, too.

One day as Jesus entered a courtyard with his friends, a woman, wearing nothing more than a bed sheet, was tossed in the street by an angry mob of men. She had been caught red-handed in the act of adultery. She was sleeping with someone other than her husband, a crime worthy of death. With stones in their hands ready to strike, they demanded, "In the Law Moses commanded us to stone such women. Now what do you say? " (John 8:5)

Without saying a word, Jesus stooped down and began writing in the sand. As he did so, all of the attention shifted from the shameful woman to Jesus and his sand drawing. Then he stood up and redefined the moment, "If you've never done something wrong, go ahead and throw a stone," then returned to the dirt. *Thump. Thump. Thump.* Stones dropped on the ground, and one by one, starting with the oldest mobster, each turned away in shame. Jesus drew a line in the sand that said, "This is as far as you go. You don't have permission to tell this woman who she is!"

Jesus not only saved the woman from certain death, but also restored her dignity and power. She was not her circumstance,   no longer defined by her past or her present predicament—she was more than what she had done. Jesus drew a line in the sand that divided her from her past and restored her power to choose a new future— one that was wide open. She could be anything she chose: A wife, a mother, an artist, a merchant—*anything.* No person, thing, choice, mistake, or failure would get to define her without her permission from this day forward. The line that he drew was her defining line, her defining moment—*her line in the sand.*

The moment I was diagnosed with cancer, I was faced with my defining moment. Never before had I faced any kind of serious illness, much less my mortality. I always had the luxury of health and youth because I was a typical young adult who considered himself immortal. I threw my body around like it would never break skydiving, snowboarding, mountain biking, eating what all I wanted and drinking plenty of beer. Illness and death were things that happened to old people, not thirty-eight year old guys. Then suddenly, without any warning, I was thrust into an epic battle for my life. Each day as I woke up I had to choose to fight for my life or give into death. It was a choice that caused everything around me to become black or white; the things that mattered most rose to the surface, while the menial tasks, which I spent most of my time on, sank to the bottom.

Cancer has completely and utterly changed the way I understand the power we have to choose how to live. The choice is really quite simple: We can sit back and allow life to happen *to* us or we can do what Jesus did—draw a line in the sand and take back our choices, take back our dignity and *choose how we will live our lives*. We don't have to play the hand we are dealt by our circumstances or accept that we have no options in the face of difficulties. We cannot allow our circumstances to define us! If we allow ourselves to be defined, a death sentence rings in our ears when we are diagnosed with cancer or are faced with difficulties—whatever shape they may take. We roll over, give up, and let our circumstances win.

Don't let them win! Don't take things at face value! We have the power to refuse to believe that our circumstances are the entire story. We can reject that a thing—a moment, a decision, a person, or even a diagnosis—has the power to define us. Those things are just that: *Things*. And they only have as much power as we choose to give them.

When we refuse to be defined by these things we become gamers and start to look for new angles, looking beyond our circumstances to see new possibilities. We become fighters and a diagnosis of cancer becomes a new birth, a do-over, a creative license to find gutsy ways to beat the disease and live life to the full. In short, we become Line Drawers.

The voices that call us in an attempt to tell us what we should believe and who we are, are many, and often they are false. My friend Steve calls these "voices from the cellar." Some are voices from the past that tell us that we are no good while others are of our failures and mistakes. And still others are voices of fear and anxiety. But all of them are dirty, filthy, deceptive lies. Line Drawers reject these voices from the cellar and the labels they attach and the pressure they put on us to shape who we are and what we believe about God, ourselves, those we love, and life itself.

Rather, Line Drawers tune into "voices from the balcony," voices that whisper love, patience, goodness, healing, and hope in our ears. There is one voice among all the voices in the balcony that gives us dignity, love, and power—God's voice. This is the same voice that Jesus listened to. Early on at his baptism in the Jordan River, God told Jesus,

> You are my Son, whom I love; with you I am well pleased.
>
> (Luke 3:22)

And guess what? God tells us the very same thing! God is madly, deeply in love with us—we are his beloved sons and daughters! And oh, how he is pleased with us! For we are his creations, his precious creations, who have been made in the very image of God! (Genesis 1:27) This is the voice we need to tune our ears, minds, and hearts into!

God's voice of love is offered to us regardless of our behavior, regardless of our mistakes, regardless of our awkwardness, and regardless of or our performance. God's love for us is magnanimous—bigger than life itself, bigger than what is or what will ever be. His love is always enduring, never ending, and complete in every way. The remarkable truth is that the Creator of the Universe loves us no matter what—unconditionally. It is this amazing, holly, perfect, unconditional love that gives us permission to stop attempting to please everyone—all those voices from the cellar. It also frees us from feeling that we have to run around like crazy trying to please God, for he is pleased with us already as we are. God's perfect, unconditional love sets us free to simply be human, no more and no less, and allows us to face challenges like cancer because his love is bigger than illness and reminds us that he is always with us. Ultimately, God's love frees and empowers us to choose how we live and whose voices we want to listen to that will shape and define who we are. It is God's loving voice that grants us the power to become Line Drawers.

Throughout my journey with cancer I have been introduced to several fellow Line Drawers. My friend Clif came to me in the hospital just after my first surgery to remove twelve inches of my colon. He walked into the hospital room gave me a chunk of asphalt wrapped in a paper bag. "What's this?" I asked, a little confused. "It's the road to recovery," he said with a smirk. Clif knew something that I didn't. He knew that tests, scans, surgeries and chemo, while not being what I wanted to endure, were going to be part of my healing process. More importantly, he taught me that I didn't need to be a passive cancer patient who just sat and allowed the medical community to poke and prod me like some sort of experiment. I could be active in my treatment, choosing to allow a community to come around to pray, support, and care for my family and me. I have come to call this community my *Army of Love*. They have become a crucial part of my treatment protocol. Clif modeled this to me when he too, fought colon cancer. He was a fellow Line Drawer who fought valiantly till the very bitter end of his life. I miss his companionship and encouragement dearly.

Sandy fought ovarian cancer, but lost the battle about a couple of years ago. In many heartfelt conversations she reminded me that being beautiful and valuable has nothing to do with what is on the outside, though she was a remarkably attractive woman. She refused to be defined by her loss of hair or her inability to work while going through treatments. She taught me that what makes me beautiful and worthy cannot be defined by circumstances, rather that I am defined by God's voice of love and acceptance, *period*. Sandy, too, was a Line Drawer.

Scotty was an eighteen-year old cancer survivor who endured more surgeries, radiation, and chemo than anyone I have known. To my knowledge he never once complained. Simply put, Scotty taught me how to fight this disease. He taught me that I am not my cancer, that I had the ability to just be my unique self, just as he was his own unique self. Scotty's will to live, to laugh, be creative and loving far outweighed his cancer. Scotty was always just Scotty, never "poor Scotty with cancer." He was a total stud, another Line Drawer whom I miss like crazy. He passed away just a few months ago.

This is a book about my attempt to become a Line Drawer during my fight with cancer. It is my effort to put into words the lessons I learned during my first year of battling cancer (I'm in year four of my battle now). In no way do I feel it is the authority on cancer or an explanation for pain and suffering in our lives, though I do wrestle with the subjects. In many ways, these topics remain a complete and total mystery to me and I have a feeling that I will continue to wrestle with them throughout my remaining days on this earth, whether few or many.

I don't know why I got colon cancer. My family has no history of it and most that get it are twice my age. The doctors have told me that my case is clinically random, meaning that there are no medical or hereditary reasons I should have it. And I hesitate to say that I got it for thus and such reason because it minimizes God's potential to use my life apart from the disease. But what I do know is if I have something to offer from my experience that can help someone on his or her journey, I'm eager to do so. Writing about my experiences, knowing that they may help others on their life journeys lessens the blow of having the disease—though not completely. I'd rather have the best of both worlds: be cancer-free and still lend a helping hand. Maybe in the next life…

The chapters in this book were taken from my blog on *www.carepages.com*, a very useful website which allows people like me to communicate with family and friends without having to have the same face-to-face conversations over and over again. It also has given people the opportunity to respond to me and offer their words of love, encouragement, and hope. What a tremendous gift this has been to my family and me! We are reminded that we are never alone, though we have felt lonely many times. The prayers, encouragements, and love we received from our wonderful friends and families all over the globe have wonderfully overwhelmed us and have become our "voices from the balcony"—indeed,

God's voice reminding us that we are loved and accepted just as we are, regardless of our struggles and circumstances. These messages have given us the power and courage to face our challenges and continually choose life over death, hope over despair, joy over sorrow, and love over bitterness.

Throughout this whole crazy season of our family's life, we have discovered we are becoming Line Drawers: People tuned into God's voice, allowing voice of love and acceptance to define us as his beloved sons and daughters over and against the pressure that cancer has relentlessly and ruthlessly applied to our lives. My prayer is that the words that follow will serve as the same reminder for you. Draw on!

Jim Coons
March 2013
Chico, CA

1 Christmas 2008

I have an amazing wife of twenty years and three incredible children. Laughter is spontaneous around our dinner table. We just giggle as we live life as a family. We love to listen to music and dance, play board games, read good books, ride bikes, go on long walks, and take wonderful vacations. We love to spend time on our boat or on the ski slopes of Mt. Shasta or Lake Tahoe. If I had a dollar for every wrestling match I've had with my kids I'd be a millionaire. That is not to say that we don't have our struggles and rough moments—we do. But overall our life as a family is really quite amazing. Emily and I often look at each other and say, "We have the best life." And it's true—we have a wonderful life together.

Anyone with young children can tell you that the most magical time of the year is Christmas. The wonder of the holiday, the gathering of family and the anticipation of getting gifts adds to the magic of the season. Christmas 2008 was no exception: Our families had traveled to Chico to celebrate Christmas with us. A few days before they arrived, I went out to a butcher shop to buy several expensive, thick steaks marinated in some secret marinade that we would barbeque for our Christmas dinner. While at the shop I treated myself to one of their famous steak sandwiches—a total gut-bomb that caused an insanely painful stomachache that lasted right into Christmas day.

I was used to the abdominal pain, though, because I'd been experiencing it for over a year, maybe even longer. I don't remember exactly when it started but continually passed it off as an occupational hazard. You see, I was a youth pastor—had been for almost twenty years, and when you're a youth pastor you end up eating like the teenagers you're with: Pizza, cheeseburgers, French fries, soda, milkshakes—pretty much anything cheap and fast and FAT. No wonder the youth of America are getting obese! We feed them like crap and tell them it is their right.

I had gone to my doctor several times and even to the emergency clinic once complaining about my abdominal pain. They took X-rays, asked a battery of questions, poked and prodded my gut, and eventually diagnosed it as irritable bowel syndrome. They encouraged me to eat more fiber and less fat and to exercise more. They also said that I needed to reduce the level of stress in my life. "Yeah, right," I thought. "It sounds like the cure for any number of things in American society. Who doesn't eat fatty food, need more exercise and reduce their stress level in this country?"

Knowing what I know now, I wish I hadn't been so cavalier and actually took their advice more seriously. But I did try... well I kind of tried. I haven't always been the most disciplined of people on the planet. I managed to eat a little better, but *In-n-Out* burgers were so good! I bought a road bike and started riding, but it was hard to find the time to get out on the road regularly in the midst of work, family, and *American Idol.* And I even switched jobs from working with teenagers to working with adults, supposedly reducing my stress level.

Unfortunately though, it was too little too late. The damage had already been done to my body. Nothing I tried brought relief from my gut pain, and as it increased, so did my anxiety. I started to entertain the thought that I might have something serious going on inside of me. I even briefly considered that it might be colon cancer, but quickly dismissed the idea thinking it couldn't even be a remote possibility. Sometimes my stomach pain was twisting, other times it was dull and constant. Sometimes it was shooting like someone was shoving a hot poker into my gut. I started to fight bouts of constipation, and going to the bathroom became like entering the ring for a fight against a stubborn, big, mean, ugly opponent. Having a successful bowel movement was cause for a silent celebration.

As I finished barbequing the steaks on Christmas day, brothers, sisters, grandparents, in-laws, children, and even a dog or two, sat down to eat our Christmas feast. We were crowded around our too-small dining room table, elbows clashing as hands reached for more mashed potatoes, gravy, butter, and thick, savory steaks. Christmas music played from the stereo, and the room was glowing the joy of the day. The kids were eager to go play with their new toys, and the adults were ready to simply drink wine and soak in the wonder of the holiday. As much as I tried to live in this magical Christmas moment, I couldn't because joining us at the table was my intense abdominal pain—my constant, agonizing companion.

The uninvited guest forced itself on me as platters of food were passed and glasses were raised in celebration. The room grew blurry as the pain became my silent focus. I finally succumbed to the pain and dismissed myself in complete agony. I was off to the bathroom to duke it out with the toilet once again.

I'm not sure how long I was gone from the table, but I do remember hearing laughing and joyful conversation as I violently released all that was in me. It wasn't any normal bowel movement either—it was more like an explosion in the toilet followed by the most fowl stench I have ever smelled in my life. It was as if death had exited my body and filled my bathroom. It hurt, it burned, it made me break out in a cold sweat. "Some freakin' Christmas this is turning out to be," I told myself. It grew worse even still as I stood up and looked in the toilet; what filled the bowl could only be explained as a reddish-brown mess. What I had smelled was a generous smattering of my own blood mixed in with Christmas dinner and that damn steak sandwich from a few days ago. My world began to spin out of control. My heart leapt into my throat. My brain went into overdrive and I thought, "What the hell is happening to me? Why am I bleeding out my ass? Why did it hurt so badly? What was wrong with my thirty-eight year-old body? Why on Christmas?" Meanwhile laughter filled the house and *I'll Be Home For Christmas* droned on from the stereo. I immediately had two more violent, bloodstained bowel movements, and then lay on my bed in a paralyzed panic. "Oh God, I have colon cancer!" was all that I could think. I just knew it. Colon cancer had crossed my mind in the past as a fleeting thought, but now it was a reality. Not how I want to remember Christmas 2008, but it is now burned into my memory for eternity.

I went in to see my doctor again immediately after the holiday and he quickly referred me to a specialist who would perform a rectal exam and a colonoscopy. Before I left my doctor's office I asked him THE question that I feared the most, "Do you think I have colon cancer?" His reply has earned him the title as my "former doctor." He said, "It's doubtful. You're too young and have no history of it in your family. I'm sure it's a ruptured polyp or diverticulitis," a condition that causes pockets in the colon that get irritated, cause pain, and even bleed when aggravated. I felt relieved by his response and because he didn't think it was colon cancer, neither did I. After all, he was the doctor, right? We are taught to trust the opinions of those people wearing white coats who carry stethoscopes around their necks. Not any longer.

I had my appointment with the specialist about two weeks later, and after his examination he couldn't find anything that would cause the bleeding either, so he scheduled me to have a colonoscopy. "Fine," I thought. "No big deal. Not really my idea of a good time, but at least we'll make sure I'm ok." Meanwhile I was still having occasional gut pain, but I wasn't bleeding or feeling anxious because my doctor was sure it wasn't cancer, and the specialist didn't seem concerned, either. What was there to worry about? I was young and strong! We were just being thorough and cautious.

The day before my colonoscopy I was at work. I remember because it was a Wednesday, and Wednesdays are the day our whole staff gathers and we talk about the big news of the week around the church and share prayer requests with each other. I let them know that I was going in for a "procedure" the next day and asked that they pray for me. We all had a chuckle because we knew that my procedure would require a camera getting shoved where the sun don't shine. We also knew it was merely a formality because I was young and healthy. It was one of those light-hearted moment shared among co-workers— no big deal. Later that morning in another meeting we continued to laugh at my ensuing procedure. My good friend and boss, Steve, laughed the hardest because he had recently had a colonoscopy and knew the routine that preceded it. He knew that starting early that afternoon I would be drinking gallons of this evil, magical liquid that would make me release every last ounce of substance in my colon. It would turn me into the "space shuttle launch on my toilet," as Dave Berry, the humorist for the *Miami Harold*, once wrote.[1]

The colon prep procedure was about as uncomfortable as I thought it would be. I pooped a lot— I mean *a lot*. Then I pooped some more. When I sneezed I would poop. When I coughed I pooped and by 10 P.M. I was exhausted and completely empty. There was nothing left inside my body—it had all been expelled due to that magical mixture that I had to drink every 10 minutes. Emily and I eventually sat down (gently) on the couch and talked about the next day's procedure. "Are you worried?" she asked. "Not really," I replied. "I won't worry until I know there is something to worry about. I think it's nothing." The possibility of it being cancer was very remote in my thinking at this point. My Christmas day scare was a distant memory, a case of mistaken diagnosis—a freak, isolated incident.

The morning of my colonoscopy, Emily drove me to the outpatient surgery center across town and as I checked in the nurse seemed surprised to see me, a healthy-looking young man getting a colonoscopy. I told her I had blood in my stool and that we were just checking to make sure that everything was ok. She was quick to get on board and play along in our "it's not anything serious" charade. I remember laying on the procedure table in the room talking with the technician about the Miami Dolphins and looking out the window. "No big deal," I continued to tell myself. "This will be over before I know it, and I'll be back at work tomorrow." He stuck electrodes all over my head and chest to monitor my body, and then administered the general anesthetic. Instantly everything went brown and fuzzy and I faded off to sleep. I remember waking up once during the procedure and groaning because of the discomfort so they quickly knocked me out again.

The next thing I remember was waking up in a recovery room, but Emily wasn't even there yet. She had gone out to run an errand. That's how casual we were about this whole thing! She wasn't even there! The nurses came and asked where she was so I gave them her cell number then faded back to sleep. Some time later I woke up with Emily and the doctor standing over me. With a very serious and glum look on his face, the doctor began to talk with us. He got straight to the point, "We ended the procedure sooner than we anticipated because we found a significant blockage in your colon."

I was pretty fuzzy from the drugs, but my heart began to race. "What's he saying?" I thought to myself.

"It appears to be a sizable tumor, and it looks like cancer," he continued. "I've done these procedures many times and I know what cancer looks like, and this looks like cancer. I strongly recommend that you have it removed surgically as soon as possible."

Without warning, a bomb went off in my head and tears formed in my eyes. I couldn't believe what I was hearing. He was confirming my worst nightmare! Was he really saying that I had cancer? It felt as though he was pronouncing me dead. What was going on? What was happening to my perfect life? It like the earth was giving way I was beginning to sink. This was easily the worst moment of my entire thirty-eight year old life.

The next thought that went through my head were the words, "For better or for worse, for richer or for poorer, *in sickness and in health*,"—Emily's wedding vows to me. I was so thankful for Emily and that whatever the hell was happening to me, I wasn't going to face it alone. I had the best partner in the world, so I reached over and found her trembling hand. As we held hands tightly, we began to cry—the first of many tears we would shed.

We couldn't believe it: *I had cancer.*

2 Change

Everything changed the moment I was told I had cancer. I mean *everything*. It's amazing how quickly life gets reshuffled and priorities change in moments like these. It's insane really, as I think about it. Plans were changed within hours as we reprioritized our lives in a matter of a few hours. I was scheduled for a trip to Louisville that next Monday: Cancelled. I was supposed to preach in church the next week: Cancelled. I was supposed to go back to work the following day: Cancelled. This became our theme for the next several months: Cancel, change, re-think, adjust, flex, sidestep, and try to breathe.

Decisions, decisions, decisions! Nobody tells you how many decisions have to be made when you're diagnosed. Who should do my surgery? What about a second opinion? What about a third opinion? Which hospital should I have my surgery at? How fast do we need to move? What should I do about work? What should we do about our children? How in the world do we tell them that their daddy has cancer? How do we explain cancer to a five-year old? What should I do about all the commitments I've made? How do we tell a church full of people that one of their pastors has cancer? How do we NOT get overwhelmed by questions and phone calls? So many decisions! They seemed to never end.

Then the emotional waves started to flood and drown me as the questions and decisions piled up. *Death*:

That's the big one. Was I going to die? Was I at peace with dying at thirty-eight years old? Never in my life did I have to face that question. I was terrified and so deeply saddened at the thought of leaving my wife a widow and my children growing up without their daddy. The pit in my stomach grew deeper and deeper with each wave that crashed over me.

Surgery: It completely paralyzed and terrified me. I had never had surgery before unless you count getting my wisdom teeth pulled when I was nineteen. I couldn't fathom having someone cutting me open and putting his hands inside my body and then removing part of my insides! How long would it take me to recover? Would I have scars all over my body? Was I going to die on the operating table? I'd heard of that happening before.

Quality of life: Ugh! What if I made it through surgery but ended up with some sort of chronic condition or compromised quality of life? Would I ever be the same physically again?

Chemotherapy: Double ugh! I had just watched my dad do chemo and it seemed horrible and there was no way I wanted anything to do with it. It seemed altogether too painful and barbaric to me. Was I going to lose my hair and become ashen and frail and look like a cancer patient? Was I going to be reduced to a mere reflection of my former self? All these questions and thoughts came rushing at me at once like a storm-driven ocean and I was drowning under the flood.

We gathered at my parents' house with my good friend and boss Steve and began sorting things out. My folk's living room became the war room: Phones were ringing, questions were being asked, tears were being shed, and plans were being made. By that afternoon we had cancelled and cleared the decks for the next six weeks. We decided to do surgery here in Chico after a lot of conversation and phone calling to several local, well-respected doctors. And between coming off the anesthesia, overcoming the gaseous effects of the colonoscopy, taking in that I had colon cancer, and making a myriad of decisions, I was exhausted. That night I took *Ambien* for the first time and I've been on a steady diet of the sleep-aid ever since. Sleep is too precious to give it over to worry and stress. I'll wean myself off it once I'm through, but I ain't done yet.

The next day we woke up and wondered what we were supposed to do the morning after we were told I had cancer. They didn't give us a guidebook to follow. It was a make-it-up-as-we-go experience. For the first time we were faced with a huge decision: Were we going to carry on with our lives or be paralyzed by fear waiting for the cancer to overtake us? Were we going to give in to the worry and anxiety or take a step forward into the day we had before us though it seemed uncertain and terrifying? In short, *were we going to live or die*? We made a key decision that day:

We choose to live.

We drew a line in the sand and said, "Cancer is not the truest thing about our lives. We refuse to let it define us and determine our decisions. We choose life and light and we reject death and darkness." Even though we drew that all important line, we struggled, were immobilized by our fear, and felt like there wasn't a light for miles and miles. For the most part, Emily and I felt dark, lonely and horrified. Fortunately, though, we were aware of the question put before us: live or die. We chose to live, our definitive line in the sand.

It was a bitter cold and rainy day, and the forecast called for snow in the low foothills near our house. "Let's go to the snow," I said spontaneously. So we did. We called some close friends, loaded up in our SUV, and went and played in the snow. The flakes were huge and the drifts of snow were deep. We went sledding, threw snowballs at one another, and drank hot chocolate. It felt so *normal*, but a surreal dark cloud hung over us. We kept looking at each other saying, "Can you believe this? What the world is going on? What is happening to our charmed, wonderful life?" Even though we drew that vitally important line in the sand (or snow, as it were), we had lots of questions, doubts, and fears. We couldn't escape feeling that I was simply too young to have colon cancer.

Life wasn't supposed to be this way! I never considered where bad things came from prior to that day—but along with everything else in my life, this notion began to change. I had a deep sense that a grave injustice had been committed. I felt that the world had turned against me and I was its unsuspecting victim. Where did this cancer come from? Why did it choose me? What had I done to deserve it? Answers to these questions eluded me. They played hide and seek with my mind, not only that snowy day, but throughout the coming weeks and months. I still haven't found satisfying answers to them, but I concluded one thing: *God did not create cancer.* I think it crept into creation sometime after Adam and Eve ate the frickin' apple and the world fell into sin and darkness. My good friend and pastor Gaylord says, "Cancer is not part of God's plan—that's why we cut it out." Amen, brother! This, too, was an important line in the sand for me to draw because it separated God from the evil that takes place in the world. God is the giver of *good* things, not bad. He's the Author of *Life*, not the giver of death. God gave his son Jesus so that we could have *abundant life* (John 10:10), not death and despair. I couldn't see how God had anything to do with cancer other than to love me and be with me through the experience. He hasn't let me down yet, and He has walked with with me faithfully. I've experienced his love in bucket-loads since that first snowy day.

That night we continued adjust to the changes as we drove to be with Emily's family. We kept on moving, partially because we didn't know what else to do, and partially to dodge the diagnosis. When we arrived at their house, we sat and embraced each other for a long, long time. We were all in a state of shock. My father-in-law, a man of few words, looked me in the eyes and shook my hand. He told me he would be praying for me, a gesture of pure love. My sister-in-law offered me her breast milk (she was nursing their baby at the time) because a study in England showed that breast milk killed cancer cells. Now that is love at a whole new level!

The Tour of California bike race was starting in Sacramento the following morning and we had planned all along to go watch it. Ironically, the main sponsor of the race was *Amgen*, a company at the forefront of cancer drug research and development—in fact they produce a drug that I would later use during chemotherapy, though I didn't know it at the time. The city blocks surrounding the racecourse were full of cancer-related information booths. It totally overwhelmed me so I told Emily, "Don't make me go into those booths." I wasn't anywhere ready to count myself as a cancer patient yet. I wasn't comfortable with the disease and I'm still not.

Along my journey, it seemed like God knew I would be faced with insurmountable changes and obstacles so he provided inspiration and hope in big doses. We didn't realize when we were making plans to see the bike race that I would be diagnosed with cancer two days earlier, nor did we know that weekend would mark the comeback of Lance Armstrong to professional cycling. For years, Lance Armstrong has been one of my greatest heroes and inspirations. I had read about his fight with cancer and learned from him how to face challenges and obstacles with strength and determination. He taught me how to keep on living in the midst threats and hardships. Lance Armstrong is a serious Line Drawer.

Now, suddenly, Lance's story and my story were colliding in the streets of Sacramento. It was inspiring to witness his comeback and we came to refer to him as "inspiration in Lycra." Seeing him in person and knowing his attitude and his fortitude infused me with a new hope. I cried like a baby as he rode in the streets around our state capital buildings. He wasn't just racing for himself and he wasn't even racing for faceless, nameless cancer patients—he was racing for *me*. He didn't know me from Adam, but he was racing for me. With each pedal stroke I felt courage building up inside me and inspired to fight, climb, and reach for the cancer finish line. One day I hope to meet the guy and give cancer the middle finger in a photo together. I'll hang it center focus on my office wall, even if it offends the good church people. I don't really care. Cancer sucks and I'll tell it to screw-off to anyone who asks. I hate the disease and the horse it rode in on. Without asking or any kind of warning, it rides in and turns your life, your plans, your family, your finances, your job, your emotions, your spiritual life, your friendships, your body (big time) and your soul upside down. It doesn't play fair and I don't like it. It can take a friggin' leap off a cliff and die and I wouldn't bat an eye. Cancer can go back to hell where it came from and I'd be happy and laugh all the way home. I would love the opportunity to celebrate that sentiment with Lance Armstrong in a photo someday.

By the way, I think Jesus, the original Line Drawer, is giving the cancer the middle finger, too.

3 The Truest Thing

February 13, 2009

> Don't let the world around you squeeze you
> into its own mould, but let God re-mould
> your mind s from within, so that you may
> prove in practice that the plan of God for
> you is good, meets all his demands and
> moves towards the goal of true maturity.
>
> -Romans 12:2 (Philips)

I have cancer. I have a tumor in my colon. Even
though this unwanted foreign invader is growing inside
me it is not the truest thing about me, though my
thoughts and fears would have me believe otherwise. As
I thought about the fact I have cancer, my thoughts
drifted to C.S. Lewis' *The Lion, The Witch, and the
Wardrobe.* At the climax of the book the White Witch kills
the Christ-figure, Aslan, on the Stone Table. The fact that
he was killed wasn't the truest thing about him, though.
In the moment of his resurrection he reminds Susan and
Lucy of a deeper truth,

> "It means," said Aslan, "that though the
> Witch knew the Deep Magic, there is a
> magic deeper still which she did not
> know. Her knowledge goes back only
> to the dawn of time. But if she could

have looked a little further back, into the stillness and the darkness before Time dawned, she would have read there a different incantation. She would have known that when a willing victim who had committed no treachery was killed in a traitor's stead, the Table would crack and Death itself would start working backward."[1]

There was a "Deeper Magic from Before the Dawn of Time" that was at work that the White Witch didn't know about. That deeper magic was that he was the Son of the Emperor from across the sea. Aslan had a deeper identity, a deeper truth about who he was and the love in which he lived, that brought him new life.

Cancer is trying to press me into its mold, making me a "cancer patient," helpless and dependent on others. There are days when I play the "C" card and complain that I can't do it, can't make it. I give in and believe that I am helpless, a victim. My prayer has been for God to give me the wisdom and strength to proclaim my identity as his Child. That's what will help me get through these helpless moments. Of all the things that we can choose to be, choosing to realize that *God chooses us* as his sons and daughters is the greatest gift. It frees us from being helpless victims—it becomes our strength. It frees us from disease—it becomes our healing, even if we physically don't get better. It frees us from expectations—we are accepted for who we are. It frees us from pretense—we don't have to prove ourselves to God because he already loves us. Being a child of God allows us to simply be ourselves, no less, and no more.

Thanks be to God that there is a deeper magic at work here! Will you join me in prayer that my family and I can live in that deeper magic as we journey through this next chapter?

4 Darkest Before Dawn

February 16, 2009

I met with the surgeon today and got the pathology report that confirmed that I have stage three colon cancer. "Sonofabitch," I said out loud. I couldn't believe it, though I expected nothing less based on the colonoscopy report. It's official; I'm a cancer patient. Darkness set in.

In a haze I went to the gym to work out—what else was I to do? Ironically, I felt great. I couldn't tell I had cancer. As I lifted weights I rocked to U2's early 90's techno-song, *Lemon* in my headphones. The song talks about new days starting when it's darkest, at midnight. Those words resonated deep within me. It is so dark right now. I can't think of a worse time in my life. I have freaking cancer. I might die of this. I might have to have chemotherapy and lose all my hair. I have no idea what the future holds. I am falling through space and time in complete darkness. My arms and legs are flailing trying to find solid ground, but none is to be found. I'm groping in the midnight darkness. Thank God that the dawn always comes after midnight! I can't wait for that pinpoint of light, the dawning of a new day! Though this is not the news we were hoping for, we know that the dawn comes after the darkness.

I am faced with a choice today: Face cancer or run from it. Running from pain is the quickest way to more pain, and running doesn't solve the problem—it just prolongs it. But facing the pain, acknowledging that it is part of life, and dealing with it is the way to freedom and healing. That's where I believe the new day will begin. That's the moment when I can admit my limitations to my community, ask them to step up and care for my family and me. Likewise, I hope that this is the moment when God will meet me and give me strength beyond myself to rest, to step out of my role as pastor, trust him with my work and my whole life. Denying my illness will cause me to suffer more. But I am asking God to allow me to be sick and lead me to healing.

It is scary to face our darkness, but that is the path to the dawn of a new day.

5 God Is Bigger

February 18, 2009

    This is such a strange disease! One minute is despairing, the next optimistic, the next anger, the next sadness, and so it goes. I am a mixed bag. I am a waterworks of tears. No, I'm a three-year-old running and laughing on a playground. I'm a teenage girl in a horror flick about to be axed to death. No, I'm a flying superhero defeating aliens from outer space. I'm a wise philosopher. No, I'm a crying baby relying on my mother for my next meal. I'm a boxer on the ropes getting pummeled by a bigger, tougher, more experienced opponent. No, I'm just a fucking confused mess of a human who wants to know what just happened to his normal life.

    And today I am a lottery winner because my chest x-ray came back and it was clear. That means the cancer hasn't spread to my chest.

    Who knows what the news will be tomorrow? The hope is more good news from the abdominal CAT scan on Thursday. But it is uncertain. The results could be horrible. My guts could be riddled with cancer and I won't even know it. I may have one foot in the grave, *Taps* playing somewhere in the distance, the Grim Reaper poised to take me away this very moment. I'm suspended in mid-air between life and death, between what was and what will be. I can't return to yesterday...it was ripped from me the moment I heard the words, "You have cancer." But I can't rely on tomorrow...it's been stolen by uncertainty.

I only have today, so I choose to be thankful that God is bigger than all this garbage. No matter how bad it may get, no matter how black the darkness, no matter how tragic the news, no matter, no matter, God is bigger. He's bigger than the tallest mountain…he created the mountains. He's bigger than the deepest oceans…he created the oceans. He's bigger than the widest deserts…he created the deserts. And he is most certainly bigger than my illness…he created me, too. That's where I'm hanging my hat. That's the light that warms and guides me during this dark hour.

I am choosing to defy cancer's pain by asking people to pray. That's how I am drawing the line between the pain and me. I am determined not to let it define me. I want to be ushered into another reality—God's reality—through the prayers of the people rather than wallow in my anguish. I want to be reminded that before I was a cancer patient that I was God's child, that I was loved, that I had another purpose in life that was beyond laying in bed and crying my days away.

I'm not sure what it is about prayer that makes a difference. In many ways it is a complete mystery. I wonder if it is our faith that causes God to answer our prayers the way we want him to. Or maybe through some power of God we are fused together with what he is already going to do, so when we ask God for something it happens because it was his plan all along? I don't know. But I am trusting in its power to lift me out of the pain and bring me back into the light. Thanks for praying.

6 Bricks In The Wall

February 20, 2009

I'm realizing that there are many bricks that make up the wall of cancer. I placed one today when I had my first CAT scan. If I had a brick for every scan, probe, poke, and monitor to which I am subjected, I could build a skyscraper. There is a whole other world of cancer out there that I've been exposed to due to my diagnosis, my dad's Chronic Lymphatic Leukemia, and through others in our church and community. It's a world of subtle nods of acknowledgement between patients. They share in the fellowship of chemo and radiation. They each have sat for hours in sterile plastic infusion chairs watching bag after bag of poison drip, drip, drip into their veins. They have each been sucker-punched by the words, "You have cancer." They have been pushed to the edge of death's hallows. When they see each other and nod, there is a deep knowing, an invisible yet very real bond shared. Now I'm experiencing it firsthand. I can't say I'm glad to know about this clan because it's a family that I don't want to be a part of. But we don't choose our families, do we? They choose us.

As I lay stretched out on the CAT scan table, I couldn't help but pray for all the other people who have occupied that spot. I wondered what fears haunted them, what parts of their bodies were being attacked by mutated cells, what crying family members waited for them in the lobby. You don't end up on that table unless something has gone wrong and your life hangs in the balance. Darkness sang in the "whir" of the machine around my head as it took images of cells-gone-bad. Hope was sucked from me each time I had to hold my breath for another image. Cold sweat soaked my hospital gown. This damn machine had the power to tell me that cancer was attacking my liver, lungs, and brain. There is no hiding in an advanced imaging lab table. It is the table of truth.

Like a sunburst break in a stormy sky, I remembered something as the machine spun and took its tumor photos. God was on that table with me! He made a promise to always be my God! He told me that he would never leave or forsake me! I've always thought of God being huge and powerful—the one who threw the stars in the air and made vast blue oceans. He molded the high mountains and breathed the wide plains. But he is also small enough to make puffer fish and porcupines. He gave roses their sweet smell and stingers to bumble bees. He's big enough to make the sky, but small enough to count the hairs on my head—and to lie on the CAT scan table with me and with all those who came before. It was strangely peaceful to realize the smallness of God in such a foreign and scary place. Though truth about my body would be exposed on that table, a deeper truth found me in the lab: God is with me no matter what, in my corner, holding me upright, giving me the courage to live my life even if it is threatened by cancer.

7 Determined To Live

February 23, 2009

> What came into existence was Life,
> and the Life was Light to live by.
> The Life-Light blazed out of the darkness;
> the darkness couldn't put it out.
>
> (John 1:4-5, *The Message*)

These are words that I am choosing to live by today. I'm discovering one of the biggest battles in the war with cancer is the battle for my mind. How easy it is to get ahead of the information that I have about this disease! It's human nature to somehow expect the worst—probably the same instinct that causes us to slow down on the highway to look at accidents. So the challenge is to not get ahead of today, not get ahead of the information that I have and to choose to live in hope and in the moment I have been given.

> *Today I can't eat anything solid,*
> *but I still get to be a husband.*
> *Tonight I have to take that awful stuff to clear my colon,*
> *but still I get to be a dad.*
> *Tomorrow is surgery,*
> *but still I get to be a son.*
> *Tomorrow my journey takes a definite turn,*
> *but still I get to be a friend.*

Pray I win the battle for my mind. Pray I maintain self-control. Pray I don't go to the dark place and assume the worst. What will worrying do about it besides paralyze me and keep me from living today to the fullest?

Keep praying boldly—God can handle it.

Today, I choose to live.

8 Mysteriously Faithful

February 24, 2009

My surgery will take place this afternoon. As I'm preparing for it, I've been doing some thinking. Figuring out God is not easy! I've been trying to do it for the past couple of weeks, but I feel like I'm groping in the dark. Why does God allow cancer? Why does God allow suffering? Why does God let cruddy things happen to good people? I don't get it. And what bugs me even more is that some people get good news while others receive bad news. Like yesterday, for example: I got great news that I have only one tumor. But for others there is more than one tumor, there are inoperable cancers, no news at all—just tragedy. Does that diminish my good news? No, it most certainly does not. Good news is good news. But it does make God damn confusing. The universe and the God that created it seem more mysterious to me than ever. I can't figure it out!

So often I throw up my arms in surrender, not knowing which way is up or down. But then I remember that God has not failed me yet. He has been my faithful Savior. Like the time I was told that I should never be a pastor by a clinical psychologist. It was the hardest blow ever dealt me. I had prepared for years, spent thousands of dollars, and was certain God had called me to be a pastor—only to be ambushed and told I couldn't cut it. But God was there to catch me, prop me back up, and send me back into the ring to keep fighting. He healed me, held me, reminded me, and gave me hope. That was ten years ago. I've been a pastor for seven years.

Or the time I was diagnosed with severe depression during graduate school. God reached down, scooped me up from the bottom of the dark pit, and set my feet on solid rock again. He gave me community, acceptance of myself, and courage to face my sad feelings with grace and strength.

- When I became a father for the first time…God was faithful.
- When Emily and I struggled in our marriage…God was faithful.
- When my dad was diagnosed with Leukemia…God was faithful.
- When my best friend's dad killed himself…God was faithful.

God was faithful.
God was faithful.

During each of these events I notice that God didn't stop the tragedy. He didn't stop the pain. He didn't change the course of events that I am aware of. But he was there, he was graceful, he was loving, and he held me close. He didn't leave me. He didn't abandon me. He didn't leave me as an orphan to fend for myself against a cruel world. Not at all. He came to me, steadied me during the shaking, comforted me when I wept, strengthened me when I was weak, and loved me when I felt unlovable. He was faithful even though my universe was crashing down around me.

God is a mystery. God is faithful. Both statements are true at the same time. What a trip. What a mind-bender. What a relief. I need both today as I head into surgery. I need God to be a mystery because it allows him to still be good when my circumstances are bad. God being a mystery allows me to separate cancer from God and his will for my life. And I need God to be faithful because I am dead afraid of being cut open and operated on in a few hours. I need him to be faithful again because I am weak, vulnerable, and scared. I need him to be faithful because my future is uncertain at best, tragic at worst. I need to know I can count on him no matter what the results of surgery and the biopsy are.

Mysteriously faithful. I can live with that as I go into surgery today. I can live with that.

9 Humpty Was Pushed

February 25, 2009

The people in white and blue wheeled me into the pre-op room, this place where they line up victims on gurneys with only sheets separating them. You literally feel their anxiety through the thin space. Tears are shed, worried families gather, needles are stuck, lines on bodies are drawn, prayers and prayed, and everyone is sterile and nervous. Let me tell you, it's not a holiday destination.

The nurses are nice enough I suppose, except the one I had. She had the bedside manner of a cut-man in a boxer's corner. A jaded woman of about fifty-five, she was all-too-eager to show me what I was in for. You see, up till I was pushed over the ledge by this white-coated bully, I thought my incision was going to be small, not too invasive. But Nurse A-hole dispelled that myth with one fell swoop as she lifted her shirt to reveal a ten-inch zipper running from her sternum through her belly-button from her colorectal surgery.

Why? Why did she have to do it? As she lowered her shirt I was pushed as from the top of tree, free-falling toward the earth, slapped by branches and leaves, out of control and plummeting. What was about to happen to me? I lay there sweating, short of breath, seeing white terror sheets. It was at this moment that I realized that I had no control over my life. I went from thirty-eight to one. I was an infant at the mercy of my environment. I was pushed off the wall, out of the tree, over the ledge of my security and self-reliance and into the abyss. I couldn't save my own life. I lacked the power to affect the outcome of my surgery one iota. But then again, who of us really has the strength and ability to control our lives on any given day? No one.

I had surrendered my life to God at least a thousand times in my life: At summer camps, in churches, in moments of distress. I had made countless bargains with God: "If you get me through this, then I'll live for you!" But never, and I mean NEVER have I found myself truly out of control, staring death in the face, not knowing the outcome before this moment in the pre-op room. "God, I trust you with my life." It may be the shortest yet most earnest prayer I've ever uttered. I meant it, too.

I'd like to slap that cold-hearted nurse, but I also want to thank her. She helped me trust God in a way I've never trusted him before.

10 Good And Bad News

February 27, 2009

Why does news seem to always come in the categories "good" and "bad?" Maybe because it always seems to be true. Well, today we have some good news and some bad news.

First the good news: I'm up and about, took a shower, shaved, and I'm disconnected from the myriad of wires and tubes that I've been chained to for the past several days. Yes! I feel set free! It looks like I'll get to go home tomorrow if I'm able to eat some real food and poop. Sooooo... pray for POOP!

Now the bad news: Within a forty-minute period this morning, I had my catheter and my epidural removed, and then got the oncology report. It was like a tidal wave crushed me into the rocks. The report wasn't what we wanted to hear at all. It seems that the tumor has permeated the wall of my colon and there is evidence of tumor on five of the twenty-one lymph nodes that they removed from near my colon. What does that mean? It means that I still have this damn cancer running through my body—somewhere, everywhere it seems. Who really knows? It means that surgery didn't cure me and most disappointing of all, it means that I have to undergo chemotherapy. To what extent and for how long is yet to be determined by the oncologist after I recover from surgery in a few weeks.

The news was too much for me: I puked.

I can't believe that having my gut ripped open, cutting through all the muscles and tissues, and cutting out ten inches of my intestines didn't cure me. I'm stunned. I'm bummed. I'm pissed. I'm am deeply disappointed. I can't believe that this hell-journey isn't even close to being over. I just went from thinking I was going to be back to normal in six weeks to becoming a full-fledged cancer patient. This stuff could be with me for years to come—a lifetime even. Crap. We are now re-thinking the next several months and making space for the journey to continue. We were hoping, along with all of you, that the journey would be much shorter, but we were wrong. We are deeply sad, disappointed, and crying many tears. We are angry, too.

Immediately after those forty minutes from hell, my friend and colleague Greg prayed with me. As we did so, God descended upon us and overwhelmed us with his presence. It was so clear that he hasn't left my bedside for even a moment. Though it was a horrible knowing I still have cancer, it was also beautiful because even bigger than cancer is God's power and presence. As awful as the moment was, it was also beautiful. *A beautiful awfulness.* Oh, how grateful I am that I'm not journeying alone! God is with me—always has been, always will be.

11 Thank God For Cancer... Really?

March 2, 2009

I have a great life. It may sound strange for me to say that when you take into consideration that within a three-week span I've had a colonoscopy, been diagnosed with cancer, been run through a battery of x-rays, scans, and tests, given away all my work responsibilities, gone through major surgery, and am now at home recovering and, according to my wife, "wasting away" (i.e. losing a bunch of weight—who needs it anyway?). But really, I'm doing pretty well, all things considered.

It's been great to be home and be back doing somewhat normal things. Last night I made a bowl of cereal and it felt great to make *myself* something to eat. I'm tired of being waited on. I just want to take care of myself again like a normal person.

As I was released from the hospital on Saturday and as the nurse wheeled me out to the curb in a wheelchair, I was overwhelmed by the smell of almond blossoms and the warmth of the sun. Then, a bit later as I lay down in my own bed and looked around my room, I had tears in my eyes because I was so grateful to be home and in my own bed. It was like being born all over again. I can't really explain it to you, but I'll try...

This whole experience, as fast as it's been, seems to have always been with me, and it has changed *everything*. It's changed my relationship with Emily and the kids; the little things that used to seem so big have taken their place as truly "little." The important things have come to the forefront: Laughter, time spent with family and friends, scripture, prayer, worship and even mealtimes together. As much as I love my work as a pastor, I really haven't thought about it much, in part because I have such a great team that has picked up the load in my absence, but more so because life is much bigger than work. I haven't always understood this.

I confess that too often my life has been my work. Please kick me if I go back there after this is behind me. Yes, I need to work, but no, it doesn't need to be the sum-total of my life. When I have had the opportunity to talk with people who are near the end of their lives about what they would change, they say what I have just said: Life is about family and friends and God, not about working harder, being more successful, and making more money. And I've always said to them, "Yeah, totally. I get it."

Wrong! I didn't get it at all.

But now that I'm staring death in the face, I think I'm beginning to understand. Oh, how young I am and how much I still have to learn!

In some ways—and this is a stretch for me—I want to say, "Thank God for cancer." Did I really just write that sentence? Really? Yes, really. Not because I want cancer, don't get me wrong. But thank God for what this cancer is teaching me. Thank God for what this cancer is correcting in me. Thank God for what this cancer is doing to remind me about community, about love, about priorities, about relationships, about faith, about *myself*. I suppose it is really God teaching me, but he seems to be using cancer as the medium to teach me these hard but good lessons. Thank God that I'm being taught through my suffering.   It's strange, but not surprising,   that suffering and learning go hand in hand…

12 Evolution's Best Day

March 4, 2009

We have had a great couple of days recovering here. Each day it seems that I feel exponentially better than the last. Last night I was walking up and down the stairs in our house to try to get a little exercise and realized that I was starting to breathe hard. It felt great! But then I thought I should stop lest I start popping out staples in my belly or something crazy like that. But that is an indicator that I'm feeling a ton better than even a few days ago. I am thankful that my body is recovering as quickly as it is. I don't do idle well at all. I'm ready to get back on the bike and get my legs back under me. You can pray for patience now because it's still a long ways off.

Well, you knew this would happen sooner or later (probably sooner if you know me at all), but I have a reflection on U2's new album, *No Line on the Horizon*. It's from the song "Stand Up Comedy" which is my pick for the best song on the album. There's a line that talks about how God's love grows over time, and as we realize it, our discovery of that evolving love becomes our "very best day." As I've moved through the past three weeks in a world of emotions: Grief, anger, sadness, guilt, joy, shame, freedom, fear, pain and euphoria, something has happened in my spiritual life for which I am so grateful— I have come to realize the hugeness and magnitude of God in a brand new way.

I've always known God was big and that he created all that there is. But I'm experiencing God's bigness *for me*. While all this has been happening to me and to my family, I have been unable to maintain the spiritual practices that I was doing before this began. For example, I usually write in a journal almost daily as part of my prayer life, but now I've written in it only once in the past three weeks. Before this all happened I was reading through 1 Samuel in the Bible and I was loving it. But now I haven't picked up the Bible in weeks. Yes, I've read my Bible, but not in the regimented, disciplined way that I did prior to cancer arriving.

I am discovering that there are times, such as this, to simply rest in the bigness of God—and that is enough. There are times in life when we need to simply rest in the truth that God's love is big, and growing bigger all the time as we come to discover the height, depth, and breadth of it. And there are times in life, like this, to rest in his love and to allow that to be enough.

Praying the same old prayers to the same old God isn't adequate when you are told you have cancer, because the last time I checked, this damn disease kills people. The threat of death has a way of making one's prayer life a little louder, a little more urgent, and a little more desperate. Sometimes I don't even know how to put words to my prayers because I'm so paralyzed by fear. That's when I have to remember God's words that he hears my "groans" (Romans 8:26) and have come to appreciate the hugeness of God and his love the most. I don't have to explain myself to God—he already gets it. He gets me, my fear, anxiety, hopes, and dreams. All I have to do is... well, nothing because just acknowledging his presence is enough. He takes it from there. It's the evolution of God's love in our lives as we experience all the crap the world throws at us.

Given all that, it is remarkably liberating and wonderful to know that God is bigger than this disease, bigger than my fears, knowing that he understands that I can't have my "quiet time" right now. He's big enough to know that I can't even put words to my prayers and requests and longings. That's huge for me because it gives me the dignity to be "just me" and not a super-Christian hero or something. I'm not. I'm just Jim and I have cancer and I need a big freaking God who loves me as I am.

13 Side Steps

March 5, 2009

Last week my friend Clif visited me in the hospital. He's a fellow colon cancer patient and knows how this stuff goes down, so he offered me an analogy for how this cancer thing works. He said that most people talk about getting through cancer by taking one step at a time, but he's found it helpful to talk about it in terms of *side steps*. This is so true. Before I got the oncology report in the hospital, I was hoping that surgery was all I needed—a step forward. But then I got the news that I would need to do chemotherapy—a side step—not really a step back because it leads to recovery, but not really a step forward because it delays recovery, too. And I feel like I keep waiting for more information, side stepping, before I can take steps forward and get through all this craziness, confusion, and pain.

Today we took another side step as I met with Dr. Keech, my new oncologist. He helped us to know what this next side step would entail. Essentially I'll be starting twelve rounds of chemo later this month, hopefully ending some time in August. Each round will be approximately forty-eight hours long every two weeks. It sounds like this is normal protocol for people with this type of cancer. He said that without chemotherapy, the chances of the cancer returning are about 40%, but with the drugs it's about 15% within the first five years. The first big date will be the one-year marker because the chances of recurrence are highest this first year, and then get progressively less years two through five. So the news that I will be thinking about colon cancer, especially for the first year, and then for the next four years is another side step. Truthfully, I just wish I didn't have to think about it at all.

I'm trusting that God will meet me in the waiting, and that my side steps along with my community, this *Army of Love*, and my faith with a dash of U2 will not feel hopeless, but turn into a beautiful faith-filled dance.

I'm looking forward to getting my staples out this afternoon and spending time at the Sierra Nevada brewery with my friend Todd. I've been told that ale will cure what's ailing you. I want to test that theory for myself.

14 Talk It Out

March 6, 2009

I feel great about what the doctor said yesterday (though I still feel like he was talking about some other person and I can't believe that this is *my life* right now, but I digress). There is a 15% chance that the cancer *might* come back again within five years. With those odds, I say, "Let's go to Vegas baby!" That means that there is an 85% chance that these twelve rounds of chemo will be the end of it and we will be done with cancer forever. If, by this slim chance, the cancer comes back then that means the fight will go on longer than we anticipated. But read this: *We will fight no matter what happens.*

I am finding that a host of feelings comes with a cancer diagnosis: sadness, anger, confusion, or fear. Not only am I experiencing these feelings, but my family and friends are as well. Therefore, I encourage you to feel in the Technicolor, 3-D, unrated version of your feelings. Go for it—let those feelings flow. Talk it out. Talk to your family, your friends, pastor, counselor, pet rock, God, the universe, whatever. That is one of the main reasons this *CarePage* is such a great release for me: It allows me to get my feelings out there so they don't eat me up inside like a cancer—I hear that stuff will kill you.

Don't let it. Get your feelings out there so you don't have to carry them around like a giant, heavy burden weighing you down. Even though talking about them won't change our circumstances—cancer will still remain—it will change us and our perspective. This is huge because it allows us to draw some important lines in the sand between our feelings and who we really are. We are not our feelings—we are so much more! We are God's chosen children, making our way through this crazy, unpredictable life. So go talk out those feelings! Don't let them eat you up and spit you out. Reclaim your belovedness!

15 Hills And Mountains

March 9, 2009

The words from the chorus of U2's song "Crazy Tonight" are ringing in my ears as I journey through yet another day of cancer. The song talks about life and circumstances being mountains, not just small hills. Let me tell you this: Cancer is no freakin' hill, it's a big ol' mountain and I'm just in the foothills starting to gain some elevation. I have a long, long way to go.

This disease is as much a battle of the mind as much as it is of the body. Last night my mind was the battlefield. I keep thinking about the worst-case scenarios. In my darkest moments, especially at night, I have been anxiously wondering if I am going to die and leave my wife a widow and my children fatherless. I also fear that chemo will be awful, that I'll be throwing up uncontrollably, lose all my hair, and have that ashen, sunken look of other cancer patients. I hate this disease. It is preying on my mind, making me sweat and panic like I never have before. Please pray for my mind. Pray, along with these words from U2, that I'll "make it to the light" although that journey seems very dark today.

16 A Prayer For Today

March 9, 2009

A Prayer Based on Psalm 119

God, for today, this is my prayer. Hear my voice.
Be good to your servant while I live,
that I may obey your word.
I am laid low in the dust;
preserve my life according to your word.
My soul is weary with sorrow;
strengthen me according to your word.
My comfort in my suffering is this:
Your promise preserves my life.
In the night, Lord,
I remember your name,
that I may keep your law.
At midnight, Lord,
I rise to give you thanks for your righteous laws.

The earth is filled with your love, Lord;
teach me your decrees.
It was good for me to be afflicted so that I might learn your
decrees.
I know, Lord, that your laws are righteous,
and that in faithfulness you have afflicted me.
May your unfailing love be my comfort,
according to your promise to your servant.

Let your compassion come to me that I may live,
for your law is my delight.

My soul faints with longing for your salvation,
but I have put my hope in your word.
In your unfailing love preserve my life,
that I may obey the statutes of your mouth.
Save me, for I am yours;
I have sought out your precepts.
To all perfection I see a limit,
but your commands are boundless.
I have suffered much;
preserve my life, Lord, according to your word.
Accept, Lord, the willing praise of my mouth,
and teach me your laws.
Though I constantly take my life in my hands,
I will not forget your law.
You are my refuge and my shield;
I have put my hope in your word.
Sustain me according to your promise, and I will live;
do not let my hopes be dashed.
Uphold me, and I will be delivered;
I will always have regard for your decrees.

Trouble and distress have come upon me,
but your commands give me delight.
I rise before the dawn and cry for help;
I have put my hope in your word.
Hear my voice in accordance with your love;
preserve my life, Lord, according to your laws.
Look on my suffering and deliver me,
for I have not forgotten your law.
Defend my cause and redeem me;
preserve my life according to your promise.

Your compassion, Lord, is great;
preserve my life according to your laws.

See how I love your precepts;
preserve my life, Lord, in accordance with your love.
May my supplication come before you;
deliver me according to your promise.
May your hand be ready to help me,
for I have chosen your precepts.
I long for your salvation, Lord,
and your law gives me delight.
Let me live that I may praise you,
and may your laws sustain me.

In Jesus' Name,
Amen.

17 The Love Train

March 15, 2009

In the late 1980's U2 went on tour with B.B. King and his band. It was called *The Love Town* tour. Today, as I was coming home from beautiful Lake Tahoe, I started listening to some of the recordings from that tour. Such great rock and blues! Ah! It feeds my soul!

One of the great songs they did together is called "When Love Comes to Town," a bluesy tune that speaks of the arrival of love like a train pulling into town. It follows the story of a young man's foibles being interrupted by love's rescue. Images of Christ crucified howl as the song reaches its climax. It is a beautiful work of art.

I love the idea that love is like a train rolling into town, catching it, and measuring your life by its arrival. What did we do before *Love* arrived? How do we live in response to the arrival of *Love*? What do we do with this *Love*? How does *Love* affect us? How does *Love* change us? How does *Love* rescue us?

These days I don't know much because of the whirlwind of cancer. But I do know this: *Love* has pulled into my town. Let me tell you, it's a big train. It's a big, wonderful train that keeps on coming. I can't see the caboose; it's such a long train.

I had a horrible, horrible day the other day at Lake Tahoe (I know—it seems impossible to have a bad day at Lake Tahoe—but thanks to cancer, I did.) By the time bedtime rolled around I was shuffling around like I was a hundred years old. My legs were tired, my gut hurt, my circulation was shot, and my feet were freezing cold. I laid in bed moaning and groaning in my suffering. When Emily came to bed, she put socks on my feet because I couldn't sit up to do it myself, rubbed my toes, then held me to get me warm. I don't know the exact words I mumbled to her, but it was something like, "I give up. This sucks."

The great news is that *Love* doesn't give up, and certainly doesn't suck. As I woke up the next morning, Emily and I laid there again in the same suffering bed from the night before and named all the good things in life: Family, our friendships, a great marriage, God, hope, Lake Tahoe, new days, and love. *Love* came to town. It came steaming into the station called cancer and eclipsed the pain, the stress, and the anxiety of the disease. Thank God! Someone needed to intervene and get us back on the right track where cancer doesn't call the shots and wear us down, and that someone was *Love*.

Cancer is like a playground bully—it thinks it's all bad and bigger than me, but it's not. Cancer is insidious, attacking in the most precarious moments. It attacks not only my body, but my mind, emotions, spirit, and relationships, too. Cancer needs to be put in its place, under the weight of *Love* and I found a sure-fire way to do it: *Gratitude*. Remembering and naming all the gifts we have received in life, all that is good and right is the way to put cancer back in its box. Cancer would love to define everything in my life, but I won't let it. I am a Line Drawer, dammit! Cancer will not define my family, my friendships, my marriage, God, hope, Lake Tahoe, and new days. It will impact those gifts, but won't ever define or own them. Cancer is just too weak, and *Love* is just too strong.

18 "How Are You?"

March 15, 2009

Since being diagnosed with cancer and going through surgery, I have grown to appreciate those who resist our culturally-conditioned greeting, "How are you?" Such greetings roll off our tongues without much thought at all, don't they? Often we don't realize the implications of such greetings. For those of us who are facing cancer and so many unknowns, who are in a fight for our very lives, this question carries tremendous weight. And unless I want to be superficial and say, "I'm doing fine," be prepared to sit down for about an hour and really listen to my heart.

However, the truth is that I cannot sit down with each person that asks that question, nor do I want to. You may be the twentieth person to ask me that question in a day. So please understand if I just smile and nod, or blow you off. It's not that I don't want to talk. It's more that I don't have an easy answer or the energy for your questions. There *are* no easy answers for that question. Having cancer is complicated. It's all over the map, and the answer of how I'm doing changes several times a day as I receive new information about my disease and as I ride the emotional roller coaster caused by it. Here's the deal: *I don't even know how I'm doing.* How can I tell you something that I'm not even sure of myself? It's too much.

Here's a tip: If you run into either Emily or me, an easier and more appropriate greeting is, "It's good to see you!" This question expresses what we hope is a genuine warm greeting, makes us feel validated, but doesn't require us to bear our souls every few minutes to each person we reunite with.

I look forward to the day when I can return to our culturally conditioned greetings superficially, replying, "I'm fine. How are you?" Oh, to be back to that place again where it's ok to talk on the surface. But for now we are being pushed to the depths of our physical and emotional lives. We can't do "small talk" when we live at such depths. We don't have the time or energy for it. Thanks for flexing with us and speaking our depth of language.

19 Information Is Power

March 16, 2009

Today I went by my oncologist's office to get my "binder." It's the binder that you never want someone to hand you. It's all the information that the doctor gives you when you are about to start chemotherapy. It tells you all about the different toxins you'll be receiving and all the side effects each will cause. I have to be honest: I am overwhelmed. But I'm glad I have the binder because information is power.

We are learning quickly that cancer puts a kibosh on all sense of planning ahead. It's a very foggy disease. One minute you could be headed down one road of treatment or plans, then without warning, it redirects you in the opposite direction. No turn signals, no warnings, just a bunch of sharp U-turns and side-street-detours. So to receive information that offers a little vision of the future is empowering. It allows me to prepare, get my army gathered, and start praying in a certain direction.

The main side effects of my chemo will be fatigue, nausea, some mild hair loss, and sensitivity to cold—both to touch and taste. They say that I'll need to wear gloves to pick up anything cold and I'll need to eat and drink room temperature foods and liquids. As with all drugs, each person's response to chemo is unique, so we'll just have to wait and see what this stuff does to me. Hopefully it just kills the heck out of those cancer cells.

Today I feel like I have cancer. Cancer and I have become one. I need to discipline myself remembering that life is made up of more than cancer. But the disease is pervasive today. It's everywhere I look. It's in every thought I have, I simply can't escape its grasp. It has me against the wall, threatening me like an inner-city mugger after my wallet. It won't let me get on with life. Ugh! What a weight to carry around! It seems like every conversation and every decision is about cancer, and that this disease is choreographing every movement. Will it always be like this? I hope not. I pray not. It cannot. I won't allow it. I need to remember that I'm a Line Drawer. But today, I need the other Line Drawers to guide my hand. Help me reach down to the sand and divide me from cancer once again. We have been melded together too closely for my taste.

Help.

20 Midnight Cowboy

March 18, 2009

Last night as I was trying to sleep I began to wonder when this dream (or should I say nightmare?) will end. It truly is dream-like. My goodness, just a few weeks ago my life was so different. This thing has happened so quickly, and we've been sent on a new journey, in a new direction.

I've been through tough times before, and in some ways this is similar. During my depression in seminary the image of wandering through the desert became a metaphor for my life. I imagined myself wandering about in the dryness, looking for the occasional oasis, ultimately looking for where the desert ends and *terra firma* begins.

I have a similar image now, but it is not one of the desert—it is one of darkness. And something I've learned is that, as much as I'd like to, I can't avoid walking into the desert, or in this case, the darkness. I mean, I could, but "denial" isn't a river in Egypt, is it? Sometimes we're called to walk in the desert or to take the midnight-journey. Just call me the Midnight Cowboy, riding this cancer-horse through the darkness.

You might be saying, "Ok, this guy is definitely on serious pain meds!" But hold on, I have a point! My point is this: My experience is that running from the darkness and chasing daylight only prolongs the agony and keeps us from finding hope and the lessons and wisdom that only the darkness can teach. This is my journey and I'm *called* to walk it.

My hope, and thus my ability to fall to sleep last night is that walking into the darkness is the only way to the sunrise. I can chase daylight, feudally run from darkness all day long, but eventually it will overtake me. So my decision is to face the darkness, take the journey, become the Midnight Cowboy, and look for the dawning of the new day.

Surrendering and walking this journey is summed-up in the words of U2's song "Moment of Surrender." It speaks of surrendering one's self to something larger, something unseen—God. It plays with the idea of stepping with faith into the unknown future, trusting that God will provide all the vision we need, even if is just enough for the moment.

The task before me is to surrender to *vision*—a vision of what God is teaching me, of my life on the other side of this moment, and to not be stuck with my eyes fixed on this particular moment in time. It's having a vision of life without cancer, whether in this life or the next. I'm rejecting *visibility*—those things that I can clearly see and are most present to me, and the belief that my life is only about cancer, chemotherapy, surgery, anxiety, fear, and fatigue. I'm choosing instead to look beyond my circumstances and see what God sees: Life, love, community, hope, future, and new possibilities.

Choosing "vision over visibility" as U2 sings, draws me toward the darkness, and pulls me through it like some invisible power-source. I'm certain that this is God giving me the courage and strength to walk in the darkness. And as I do so, I'm also certain that God doesn't leave me alone, but provides his Spirit to comfort, strengthen, and guide me. He also provides traveling companions, this *Army of Love*, so many loved-ones who have saddled up next to me and refused to leave me to wander alone. Thanks for joining me and traveling in my darkness. I am never alone, even when I feel lonely.

21 Kicking Cancer's Ass

March 20, 2009

I'm starting to feel a little better today, the first time after my surgery to implant my mediport, a catheter placed under the skin in my upper chest that allows them to pump chemo directly into my arteries without having to start IV's every time I'm seen. I didn't realize how much it was going to wipe me out. Emily and I went on a great walk to the bank and then to get some coffee, and I managed to play a little baseball with Jake this afternoon. Em and I are going on a date tonight, too. It feels good to feel good, if you know what I mean.

Last night as I was doing the dishes in a flash of courage and anger, I said to myself, "I'm going to kick cancer's ass!" But as I woke up this morning I asked, "What does kicking cancer's ass look like?" I had no clue. Honestly, it was easier to just lie in bed. I didn't have the energy for anything else. My shoulder hurts, my neck hurts, my back hurts, my gut hurts, my head is foggy from the pain killers... how can I pick a fight with cancer if I'm already down for the count?

So after a quick, "Help me God!" kind of prayer, I got up off the bed and decided that for today, kicking cancer's ass looks like going on a walk. There. Take that cancer! You can't keep me in bed feeling sorry for myself, you little punk!

Kicking cancer's ass will look different each day. It's choosing to live. It's going on a walk even when it hurts.

It's not just sitting on the couch. It's stepping up and living my life, not allowing this disease to dictate my day. I don't know what kicking cancer's ass will look like tomorrow, but I want you to pray that I will take up the fight all over again each morning.

I've got a size twelve with cancer's name on it.

22 Battles vs. Wars

March 21, 2009

I'm finding that it's quite easy for me to get tunnel vision, especially while recovering from surgery. Today I think is the worst day yet. The pain is sapping my strength and I feel like a limp noodle. The medications have some bummer side effects (think plumbing). I'm worked-over. It was all I could do to walk around the block a little while ago—but I did it. I'm kicking cancer's ass, but it's kicking back pretty hard. My body and mind are the battleground for this epic war.

My good friend Rylan, who is serving in our military right now, wrote to me and said, "As I have learned with fighting in Iraq, kicking anyone's (or anything's) ass doesn't just take courage, strength, or sacrifice, although that is the first step," which it sounds like he has accomplished. "Sometimes it takes patience. Sometimes it takes humility and defeat, admitting you will lose a few battles. You have the numbers on your side, fighting to the left and right of you. In the long run you will win the war."

Today I am losing the battle against cancer. I'm discouraged, mourning the loss of my health and what I would consider normal activity and energy. I'm frustrated with what's going on with my body, and looking in the mirror is a constant reminder that this is going on—I see scars and a deflated self.

I don't wish this on anyone. I don't know what I was thinking, but I thought that I would do cancer differently from everyone who has fought this disease before me. I thought that it would be a bump in the road, not a complete detour, and I haven't even started chemo yet. I'll bet that I'm not the first person who was full of ignorant hubris as they began their cancer journey.

So today, cancer got the best of me. But thank you for the constant reminder that it won't win the war even as I am humbled by my body's lack of functioning. And as Rylan said, "Sometimes it takes patience." Would you say a prayer for patience for me? And would you pray that my bodily functions would start functioning again?

I take it from your replies that you appreciate and can handle my honesty. So thanks for letting me vent yet again. And thanks for taking this journey with me.

23 Healing Pain

March 22, 2009

Today was a good day. I almost felt normal! From going to church, to taking a nap, to having a routine headache, to going for a great walk in the park with the kids who were whining and looking at the wild flowers, to dinner at my folks' house, to going out to Ben and Jerry's ice cream, to doing chores and last-minute weekend homework, to reading at bedtime... it has been a normal day.

My pain is subsiding, my body is functioning, and my head is clearing just in time to begin chemo tomorrow at 9 A.M. My regimen will be five hours of infusion tomorrow with an overnight pump, three hours on Tuesday with another overnight pump, then a quick removal of the pump on Wednesday.

I'm actually looking forward to this, believe it or not. I'm ready to see what the drugs do and how they will affect me. I know they will cause discomfort and probably will make me feel gross, and some sort of pain, but it will be *healing pain*. I can deal with healing pain. It's the senseless brand of pain that I hate. That's the pain from surgery, or from the cancer itself, but when the pain actually brings healing, bring it on. Healing pain means movement towards ridding my body of cancer. It means forward progress in this loop-d-loop world of cancer. I'll gladly undergo pain if it means that there may be a spark of light in this dark night. Bring it on.

24 The Question

March 24, 2009

Well, two days of chemo down, twenty-two to go. I'm feeling okay, actually. Some side effects are kicking in like nausea and fatigue, and I'm sure more are to come. But again, this is *healing pain*, forward movement, killing cancer. I love the analogies all of you conjure up to describe what the chemo is doing to the cancer cells: Like a soap-scrub washing them away; like Pac-Man eating up the cancer cells; like a special-ops army seeking and killing them. I like the image of Scotty Harrington's "Chemo Sucks" t-shirts that shows a dinosaur eating the cancer. They all work for me. I just want those crappy cells out of me and for them all to die! I'm confident I am beginning that process now.

The other day I finally asked the big question. I know it's not the most helpful question to ask, but it had to be done sooner or later. And I don't really expect an answer, because I don't think there is one. But I figured that God could handle the question; he's big enough, right? So I told him if he was up to answering it, that would be fine with me. (I always give God permission to do what I ask, not that he needs it or anything, but maybe it's nice for him to know that I'm on board.)

I asked God, "Why? Why me, God? What did I do, what did my family do to deserve this suffering of cancer?

What did we do to cause this?" I don't really expect an answer. Nobody I know has received one that I know of. Lots of people share their opinions or theories on this subject, but no one knows the mind and means of God. This is the biggest question we all face, and the biggest mystery with which we must live.

The closest answers come when you, my community, let me know how these messages are encouraging you or your friends, especially those who have walked a similar path that I am on now. They are like little pinpoints of light shining through the dark cloak of cancer-suffering. Somehow when you tell me that what I am going through is helping you or others, it begins to redeem my suffering...but not all the way.

At the end of the day I think what I am experiencing, and what many of us who suffer experience, is random— purely random suffering, but somehow allowed to happen in God's will. For what reason I haven't a clue, but I do know that my suffering is a symptom of a deeply troubled and imperfect, broken world. And that, my friends is the sadness in which we live. Not without hope, mind you, but still our deep reality. We live with the hope of Christ in a sad, broken world, and the two couldn't be more different than each other, could they? What a stark contrast between them! And so to be caught in the place between hope and suffering now is brutal! I've never been more aware of the contrast between these two worlds, these two kingdoms, than I am right now.

Something that I've learned about times like this is that asking the "Why?" question is not helpful. This is a very western, enlightenment-era question to ask. But there is another kind of question that is more eastern, Hebraic: It's the "What does this mean?" question. Not so much for knowledge, but for wisdom on how to live life. "What does it mean that I have cancer? What does it mean that I am suffering? What does it mean that my family is living in this hell for this season?" I still don't have the answer, but my experience with suffering in the past is that someday, when I look back on this time in my life, meaning will emerge like flowers from ashes. Think back on your own life, and your own rough times, and see if you find this to be true.

Today I spent time with a dear friend who just returned from a *Youth With A Mission (YWAM)* mission in Thailand and India. We discussed and considered love and grace. I remarked that the grace and love by which I live today is the same love and grace I lived in two months ago, only my circumstances have changed. God's love and grace have remained constant. Thank goodness for this truth! This is the anchor in my storm! God's grace is all that I have found, and it's enough. God may not answer the "Why?" question, but he has spoken definitively in history and to me personally about his meaning: *Grace.* And that is enough.

25 The Fog Is Lifting

March 26, 2009

Several months ago a friend of mine and I were talking about change, mostly because I suck at change. He gave me a great analogy. He asked, "Jim, if you are caught in one of those famous North Valley tulle fogs while driving on Hwy 99, what do you do? Do you speed up or slow down?" Duh. Slow down, of course. He asked, "Why would you do any different in change?" Good question. Change is like a tulle fog: Disorienting, confusing, and a little dangerous. When we enter into it we're never certain exactly where we are. Change is confusing. And, unfortunately, change is constant. Dang.

Chemotherapy has brought change. It is full of unknowns, uncertainties, dangers, like a thick, tulle fog settling around the unfortunate chemo-recipient. I have been in "chemo-fog" this week. It's gone well overall, but I have never felt so fatigued since the last time I did an all-night Junior High lock-in (and I swore those off years ago!). I've mostly found that sleep, a nice massage, lots of water, soft, lukewarm food, some good anti-nausea drugs, and season 2 of *The Sopranos* have been the "cocktail" of choice to manage the week. I agree with my friend and fellow line-drawing cancer patient, Scotty, on this one: Chemo sucks.

But tonight the fog is lifting a bit. I slept the afternoon away, drank a protein shake (okay, it was a chocolate peanut butter milk shake, but it sounds better to call it "protein"), and one-arm wrestled my son to the ground (the left side of the bod is still out of commission). Yes, life is regaining a sense of normalcy tonight.

Please keep me in your prayers as we head into the weekend. I'm going back to work on Sunday morning, assisting in worship services at church. It will be great to be back "in the saddle" so to speak. I've found that feeling ill can cause me to become so self-focused. And I know I'm created to serve and love others, so doing so on Sunday morning will be life giving, I'm sure of it.

26 I Like It!

April 3, 2009

For whatever reason I have felt extremely clear-minded and sharp this week. I've felt positive, energetic, hopeful, and productive. I've felt available to others, eager to help and serve, and even patient in some hard moments. I've even had some moments of wisdom that have surprised me. And I've had some amazing conversations over coffee and lunches. I don't entirely know what it is, but I like it!

At first I thought it was the steroids that they pumped into my body last week that were making me more alert and focused. That very well could be part of it. Then I thought it was the break I've had from work, letting my mind focus on something completely different. That also could contribute to what I'm experiencing. It could also be the euphoria of my nephew, Travis, being born. Certainly that factors in too.

But here's what I really think: I think God has grabbed hold of me in a whole new way because of cancer. When you have to deal with the threat of your death, it clarifies a lot. It forces you to examine your priorities and values and to make some changes.

I've been reading a well-known and received book, especially in the Chico area, called *Cancer: The Adventure of Your Life!* by Teresa K. Matthews. I have to admit that when I first heard this title a few years ago right after my dad was diagnosed with Chronic Lymphatic Leukemia, I was put-off. I thought, "Yeah, right! Nice title. It's not the happy-go-lucky adventure of a life. More like 'The Adventure of Suck' if you asked me." Oh how wrong I was! I was so confident, so smart before. I'm much dumber now. I don't assume to know a thing. The world is way more ambiguous, way more precarious, and way more mysterious now that ever.

In the book, Matthews talks about the shock of the cancer diagnosis, which is more dreaded than just about anything else in a person's life. She writes, "In point of fact, you are going to die. So is everyone else in this world! The difference is that now you see death as a personal threat, rather than a vague, mysterious concept that applies to others but not you. When you hear the word 'cancer', it galvanizes you to respond."[1]

So true, so true. This diagnosis changes you. It changes everything. It changes plans, hopes, fear, routines, relationships and conversations, prayer, worship—it changes *it all*. There is no part of my life that is not touched by cancer. It has crept its way into every nook and cranny of my being and it has changed me. But the strange thing is that a lot, in fact *most*, of this change is good. Whoa! It's that weird? I think it is, but I like it and I'm glad it's happening to me because it is making me a better person. I really believe that.

God is like a judo master. He's taking the momentum of my cancer-enemy and using it against him (my cancer is a boy if you were wondering). It's the coolest thing. What makes survivors such amazing and strong people is that something inside them (God) uses the negativity of cancer against cancer itself in order to defeat cancer. For whatever reason I feel that God is doing a work in me to help me avoid becoming a monster in the midst of this monstrous disease. The ultimate judo move!

The kids are on Easter Break now, which means we'll have lots of time together. I'm looking forward to it. But it's a bummer that I'll start another round of chemo in the midst of it. Yesterday Eliza Kate, our five-year-old, asked me where I go to get my "medicine." I told her I go to the doctor's office and I explained a little bit about it. She said that she would like to come see where I get it. So I think I'll have her visit me during infusion this week. The kids have weathered this whole thing so well. It helps that they have walked down this road with Grandpa Steve recently, too. Chemo is a household word. Kind of a bummer that it's that way, but this is the world in which we live. Cancer is epidemic—it touches or will touch each of us in some way. Statistics tell us that one in three people will have cancer, so talking about it candidly with our kids is vital. It is part of our lives, just like school, friendships, and summer vacation. Cancer is the "new normal" around our house. We have to talk about it in order to keep us from letting it control us, scare us, or kill us. Keep praying for us as we have these daily conversations in our home.

27 Taking The Risk

April 7, 2009

Risk taker. That's who I am this morning. I got a great night of sleep and woke up refreshed. Emily and I had a great morning, prayed together for the day, drank some lukewarm coffee and water (everything needs to be lukewarm because hot and cold are like fire in my throat due to the *Oxaliplatin*—the most toxic of my chemotherapy drugs), did some meaningful work from the couch, went walking with one of my former high school students, ordered a new fly-reel for the upcoming fishing season, and even took a short easy ride on the bike trainer. I'll be damned if I'm going to let cancer and chemo dictate my life. Don't get me wrong; I'm not going to overdue it. I'll rest the remainder of the day. But my mornings are good and I'm taking advantage of them. Carpe Diem!

Last night as I was struggling with feeling crappy, so I put in my good friend Andrew Burchett's new CD *Proof in the Mirror.* He describes the album this way, "If worship songs are what we sing to God, these are the songs God sings back to us." So as I sat in bed, crying and listening having one of those "I can't believe I have cancer moments," God met me in Andrew's music. One song in particular resonated with me. It's called "Place at the Table,"

I will see you through
I will be fighting by your side
When you're wounded and alone
I will carry you home
So I choose you
Will you stand for truth?
Welcome to the table courageous one
Welcome to a place reserved for you my son
O, Come to the table
I know that you're able
O, come to the table my son[1]

It's an invitation for me to come to the table that
God has set for me, my eternal home, my true home.
And the promise is that God will see me through, won't
ever leave me, will carry me when I'm a mess, and will
empower me to fulfill my destiny, even if that includes
cancer. In that way, I guess, God is redeeming my cancer
and suffering. That's how big God is! He can redeem
even the darkest parts of us and somehow, mysteriously,
allow those things to be wrapped up in his will in our
lives. So strange yet so beautiful.

Then today as I had an amazing talk and walk with
my good friend Rachel, we talked about the vastness of
God's will. We agreed that in reality, the majority of
God's will is pretty-well laid out for us: Love God, love
people, be in community, love the poor. But within those
things there is a lot of latitude. It could look a thousand
different ways and yet be all within God's will. How
freeing is that? We don't have to get hung up on trying to
figure out the perfect plan for our lives! And again, this
can also include cancer. I guess if there is a lesson that
I'm learning this week it is just how big God is. I'm

realizing that not only the good, but also the bad, are somehow, gratefully, wrapped up in God's sovereignty. Does that make God a sadist? Only if he *causes* the crap. But I don't think he does. He certainly *allows* it for some reason, maybe because, as C.S. Lewis wrote, "…God whispers to us in our pleasures, speaks in our conscience, but shouts in our pains: it is His megaphone to rouse a deaf world."[2] God wants our full attention. Let me tell you, He has mine! It is truly amazing how this disease is deepening my relationship with God.

As Rachel and I talked about all this, I said that for the past month or so I have never felt closer to God, but not necessarily through reading scripture. I just haven't read the Bible that much. But boy, the scriptures that I've read over the years are right with me each moment in my memory. I guess that's why we read, study, and pray during the calm seas of life—so that when things go crazy-stormy and get drowned by it all, we can draw on that reservoir of wisdom and relationship and assurance of faith. The scripture that came to mind for me today is from John's gospel,

> Some time later, Jesus went up to Jerusalem for one of the Jewish festivals. Now there is in Jerusalem near the Sheep Gate a pool, which in Aramaic is called Bethesda and which is surrounded by five covered colonnades. Here a great number of disabled people used to lie—the blind, the lame, the paralyzed. One who was there had been an invalid for thirty-eight years. When Jesus saw him lying

there and learned that he had been in this condition for a long time, he asked him, "Do you want to get well?"

"Sir," the invalid replied, "I have no one to help me into the pool when the water is stirred. While I am trying to get in, someone else goes down ahead of me."

Then Jesus said to him, "Get up! Pick up your mat and walk."

(John 5:1-8)

A few of things hit me:

1. The dude was thirty-eight... okay, that's freaky. I'm thirty-eight and I'm *like* that guy!
2. He's sick... okay, that's an easy connection, too.
3. Jesus "*saw* him" and "*knew*." Wow. Think about that for a second. He *sees* us and he *knows* us. Sometimes my prayers go something like this, "God, you know... ," and that's enough.
4. Then Jesus asked *the* question: *"Would you like to get well?"* It's an offer of healing. We have to ask for healing because the offer is there. So I asked Rachel to pray for my healing today, as I do for myself each day. Keep asking for my healing and the healing of others. It seems that Jesus is offering it up here.
5. The man made an excuse, "I can't get into the water!" But Jesus didn't buy the excuse, "Stand up, pick up your sleeping mat, and walk!" and he did. Bam! Just like that he was healed. I don't know if this is how it will work with me, but that's

okay, I'm open to however Jesus wants to heal me.

6. I'm *like* this guy, but I'm *not* him too. Jesus healed him. I pray he does the same for me, but that was then and this is now. Yet I read these words and am offered hope.

It's good to be reminded how Jesus works and to be given a model for how to approach him during times like these. I think boldness is the key. Don't make excuses, but cast it out there and see what you'll catch! Take a risk.

You know, my oncologist has never told me what stage cancer I have. I think it's like stage two or three since it hit my lymph system, but I don't really know. I've thought about asking him, but I've decided that I don't want to know. Here's why: *It doesn't matter to me.* Either I'm going to beat it or I'm not. Either I'm going to survive this ordeal or I'm going to die from it. But do you see the point? I'm taking a risk, because every day is a risk. Either we're going to live sold-out to life and God's will as I described above or we're not. There's not really an in-between in my mind these days. Either we're going to choose to love God, love people, be in community, and serve the poor or we're not. It's bold living. Either we're going to live each day boldly or we'll live each day in fear (of cancer stages, of our past, of our mistakes, of our past hurts, etc.) We can be like this guy who made excuses of why he laid there on his mat, or we can get up, roll up our mat, and walk home.

That's what I want to do. I want to take the risk, take up my mat and walk home. That's why I was up and on the bike again today, why I met with Rachel and walked a mile. Why I had lunch with my colleagues and planned worship and talked life. That's why I showed up late to my infusion appointment yesterday—because I was online buying U2 tickets at 10 A.M. (whoo-hoo!). I'm not letting cancer or chemo dictate my life. That's why I am writing. It's me choosing to live in spite of unknown cancer stages, infusion pumps, surgeries, and the threat of death. I am drawing a line in the sand and it feels good.

28 It's Hard To Have A Bad Day When...

April 10, 2009

It's hard to have a bad day when your new, rare U2 album shows up in the mail.

It's hard to have a bad day when your new fly-reel shows up right behind your new U2 album in the mail.

It's hard to have a bad day when your kids get to play with their great friends from Seattle.

It's hard to have a bad day when you feel like you can drive a car again.

It's hard to have a bad day when the sun is shining and you get to sit outside instead of on the couch or lay in the bed.

It's hard to have a bad day when you feel like you are emerging from your "chemo cocoon" and you realize that there is more to life than just haze.

It's hard to have a bad day when you read back over your previous *Care Pages* messages and you realize how many people are pulling for you.

It's hard to have a bad day when you realize that naps are God's gift, not something that make you miss out on life.

It's hard to have a bad day when it's the Friday before Easter Sunday, and you know that is the day that changes EVERYTHING for ALL TIME—the day Jesus died so you can have new life.

So, that being said, I'm not having such a bad day today (don't ask about yesterday, please—it wasn't so good!) But today is a new day and I'm looking forward to a good weekend, restoring health, and the celebration of the resurrection of Christ on Easter.

29 God Moves In Mysterious Ways

April 11, 2009

We coined a new term in our house: *canation: Noun*, def. a cancer vacation.

Today is a *canation*. I woke up feeling like a human being again. It's really amazing, once the chemo wears-off my head begins to clear, I get really hungry (last night it was Taco Bell!!!) and I crave exercise. I woke up early today, read John 13-19 and got back on the bike trainer. It felt wonderful to move the bod! Then, after two months of him asking, I took Jake fishing with my dad and our good friend Wayne. It was awesome! Jake was set free to be a kid, to explore, look at turtles, and get some dad time. The highlight, by far, was when he caught a fish on the fishing pole he made from a stick! What a stud! And every fishing trip has to end with a good hamburger, so we swung by *In-N-Out* and told fishing stories. Ahh, I love these *canations*!

It really is curious how this cancer causes not only physical but also spiritual ebbs and flows. It's a wild thing. It is a mystery how it happens. I was reminded of the mystery of it all today listening to U2's "Mysterious Ways" from their early 1990's album *Achtung Baby*. It's a song about John the Baptist and Salome', the daughter of Herod's wife who danced before Herod at his party just before John was beheaded (Mark 6:14-29). As with so many U2 songs, "Mysterious Ways" has more than one meaning. It appears to be a song about a dancer, but it is also about the Holy Spirit moving mysteriously, using a man's life that appeared to be a tragedy to do amazing work. As awful as John getting beheaded was, look at the impact of that man's life, at the example of faith and courage he was. I love that John didn't totally understand who Jesus was and asked, "Are you the one who was to come, or should we expect someone else?" (Matt 11:3) But God used him mightily anyhow. He helped prepare the way for Jesus, helped till the ground of people's hearts so they could hear and encounter Jesus in a way that changed their lives forever. It's a mystery that his life was used in such profound ways and yet was met with such tragedy.

I was again reminded of this mystery as I read Jesus' words at the end of John 14 this morning. He was encouraging his friends just before he was arrested. He was talking about the fact that evil (call it Satan, the Devil, or Lucifer or 'Lucy' as my friend Anthony likes to say) was coming into the world. Then Jesus says the most mysterious thing about Satan:

> …but he comes so that the world may learn that I love the Father and do exactly what my Father has commanded me.
>
> (John 14:31)

Whoa! The judo-master is at work again! He somehow allowed evil to come so that the world would know about his love for God. We see Jesus' love most clearly in His crucifixion. Evil most certainly thought it had won when the Son of God died that day. But his death wasn't the end of the story. God did a mysterious work, he worked in a mysterious way as Jesus defeated death, rolled back the gravestone, and ruined evil's plans once and for all. What the Devil meant for bad, God turned to good. Talk about a mysterious way!

I am finding this to be deeply true with cancer. This is an awful disease. It appears to be so evil on so many levels: Physical, mental, emotional, spiritual, and relational. Its threats are paralyzing. It is a hope-sucking, life-draining plague that plays dirty, striking at the heart of its victims.

But that isn't the end of the story. Amazing fruit comes from cancer. Lives are renewed, relationships are healed, words and acts of love flow easily, God becomes powerfully present, eyes are opened, and hearts are softened. God moves in mysterious ways through cancer. What Evil intended for bad, God uses for good. This is one of the craziest acts of redemption I've ever experienced. Who would have thought that cancer could be so good?

I am so glad for this redemptive, mysterious adventure with cancer. I wish like mad that it didn't include some of the discomforts and life-threats, but on the flip-side, I am thankful for these *canations*, for beautiful U2 songs, fish caught on sticks, laying in a hammock with my kids, watching the wind blow gently in the treetops, and soaking in the deep ocean-blue sky. This adventure is making me notice and absorb life as I never have before.

30 Found

April 15, 2009

As I've talked with people over the past few weeks, I've got the sense that some, not all, but some people expect me to be bitter, angry, upset or otherwise pissed-off with God, life, or the universe about what is happening to me. I've certainly asked, "Why?" and I've certainly been upset that 2009 has suddenly been hijacked by cancer. But I haven't felt the need to blame God or rage at him. I'll certainly do my best if and when the time seems appropriate, but I haven't been brought to that place as of today.

Rather, I have never felt closer with God than I have over the past two or so months. Let me see if I can explain why: There have been two major moments (and probably two-hundred minor ones) that have absolutely convinced me that God is near me, that Jesus is solidly with me, and that his loving-kindness is sustaining me. The first was the night before surgery on February 23. It was as I was doing the "bowel prep" routine (i.e. drink "super colon blow" in liquid form) that I received the news from the surgeon that my CAT scan showed only one tumor. It wasn't so much that I felt God's presence because I was spared more tumors, it was that out of nowhere the Spirit of God came and found me in such a powerful yet gentle and loving way at the most stressful moment of my life. If ever I needed to know that God was real, it was that evening. I can't remember the exact sequence of events, but I do know that as I was doing my bowel-prep business that I was worshipping the living God. My "throne-room" became God's Throne Room and Jesus found me. I literally worshipped God as I did the prep. I was wrapped in God's presence.

The second moment came later that week on Friday morning as I was recovering from my colon bypass surgery in the hospital. By "chance" (yeah, right, there aren't coincidences in God's economy!) our dear friends and colleagues Greg and Laura, both my parents, and Emily were with me in the hospital room when my surgeon came to tell me the pathology report from the specimen they had removed from me. Again, I can't remember the exact order of things, but within about a thirty-minute window of time I was told I still had cancer, that I would be doing chemotherapy, and then the epidural and Foley catheter were removed from me (not my finest hour of life). I literally threw up. But again God found me. I don't know how else to explain it except that God found me. He came right into that hospital room, right in the middle of it all, in my sadness, in my emotional pain, in my stress, in my disbelief, in my anger, in my loss, in my disappointment, in my physical pain and found me. God, in the most amazing way, reached out and wrapped me in his grace and found me. As others stepped out, Greg and I prayed and worshiped the Living God, because when God is in the room you have no other option.

Because of those two moments and many others like them, (like through your prayers, your notes, gifts, meals, etc.) I have never felt closer to God than I do today. So to answer people's question, "How are you doing?" I say, "Amazing. Never been better. Closer to Jesus than ever.

More in love with my wife than ever. More in love with my kids than ever. More fulfilled in my work than ever. More alive than ever. More clear than ever. More convinced that relationships with God and people are the most important things than ever."

In other exciting news, I'm starting to lose my hair. It's not in big chunks or handfuls, but it is definitely happening. I hear it will probably just thin and that I probably won't go bald. But every time it comes out it is a reminder that I have cancer. It first started on Easter morning in the shower. Then today, as I toweled-off my hair after the shower and I saw a bunch of hair in the towel, I murmured, "Well, I guess I need to make friends with this new reality, but I don't have to like it." There certainly are worse things to deal with. I can live without hair. In the big scheme of things I guess it's not that a big deal—it's just *hair*. But it is also a part of me. It's part of my identity, another thing that cancer would rape from me. Loss is loss, even if it's just hair. And as I've learned, all loss leads to some level of depression and grief. Yet another thing I need to adjust to in my new reality. I just wish I could get the kind of chemo that would make me just lose my back hair! Now that I could deal with!

31 Gone Fishin'

April 17, 2009

After a great week of work, exercise, and feeling mostly normal, my dad and I headed out to the lower Sacramento River for a day of fishing with Ryan Johnston. Ryan is a great guy who is a fishing guide and married to Bonnie who works with college students at our church. Not only did we get into some good fish, but also got a chance to float down the beautiful lower section of the Sac just above Red Bluff. It's a beautiful section of the river with lava rock canyons, lots of wild life, and some great fish.

One of the cool things about the day was to hear Ryan's heart to offer people hope through fly-fishing. In fact, he just started a non-profit called Cast Hope (*www.casthope.org*). The idea is to offer the platform and experience of fishing to kids who may need some hope, some fun, and an opportunity to learn to fish. I can see how this could be a wonderful gift for kids with their mentors. My mind started racing full-tilt with the possibilities that something like this could achieve in a person's life. I know that there is no better place for me to be than on a fishing stream, listening to the water, pursuing that strike from a fresh rainbow trout, experiencing the thrill of the catch, and then doing it all over again. That's what I experienced today.

Fishing gave my mind a chance to let go of all the thoughts of cancer, of all the anxiety of chemo, and even the regular stress of life. All that stuff seemed to wash downstream with my fly-line. It was definitely a vacation from cancer, or a *canation*, as I like to call it. I was "cast hope" today! Unfortunately, though, the end of the day brought on some chemo side effects and I'm, let's say, "sidelined" near the bathroom this evening. Oh well, at least the majority of the day was worry-free.

As I mentioned in my last blog, Emily and I decided that we wanted to meet with my oncologist this week. I had some specific questions for him, the chief question being about what stage my cancer is. I know I said before that I didn't want to know, but after going through a couple of rounds of chemo and after some time, I felt ready for that information. We both needed to hear the straight truth about where we stand with this cancer.

I was told that I have stage three colon cancer. Stage three because of the size of the tumor and the number of lymph nodes that tested positive as proportional to the total number of nodes they removed and tested (five of twenty-one). That is about what I predicted, so it wasn't really a shock. I'm okay with this diagnosis because even if it was better or worse, I'm still either going to live or die. And I'm still planning on kicking cancer's ass. Nothing has changed there.

I also wanted to know about the possibility of slowing down my chemotherapy treatment so as to give me another good week in-between treatments. I've so enjoyed feeling healthy, exercising, working, parenting, husbanding, and fishing and therefore wanted to see if I could do more of that, hopefully with the same net result of killing this cancer.

I was told, "No." I hate being told no! The upshot is that it is not in my best interest to slow down the treatment schedule. The data is that I have an 85%

chance that this cancer will not reoccur again in the next five years, at which point the likelihood of it ever returning is almost nil; this is based upon the treatment regimen I have been on. So if I elected to slow down treatment, I would essentially become a lab experiment because there is no data to support slowing down treatment and no way of knowing what the end result might be. Of all the things I don't want to be, a lab rat is at the top of my list, especially when my life is at stake.

Finally, I needed him to redefine "chemotherapy" for me because my earliest impressions of it were in 1986 as I watched my Grandma Coons die of breast cancer. She suffered through chemo. It seemed so barbaric, lethal, and raw. I have memories of her looking and seeming at the edge of death—she was constantly ill. So as I've anticipated my chemotherapy, I've been assuming that it will be just as awful as my grandmother's experience. The amazing, miraculous news is that the advances in chemotherapy drugs, even within the last five years, make what I am receiving completely different and more effective than what my Grandma received twenty-three years ago. It is simply amazing how effective these drugs are now compared to then, and how they can manage many of the terrible side-effects with other drugs, steroids, vitamins and supplements. In other words, we are talking about apples and oranges, totally different chemotherapies. I needed to hear that.

So today my spirits are high though my body is lacking. I'm looking forward to a restful evening and a new day and the adventure it will bring.

32 The Gloves Are Off

April 20, 2009

Today as I started round three of chemotherapy I decorated a luminary for the *Relay For Life* in honor of my Grandma Coons who died of breast cancer in 1986. I decided to put some quotes on the luminary that reminded me of her—you know, things that I remember her saying or quotes from around her house: "Be careful how you live, you may be the only Bible people read." "Amazing Grace, how sweet the sound, that saved a wretch like me," from the hymn we sang at her memorial service. "Hot damn! It's Christmas!" from the apron she wore each Christmas. I remember her rushing out of the house to our car to greet us on Christmas day with a giant smile and saying, "Ooooohhhh!" because she was so excited to see her family.

My Grandma Coons was an amazing woman. She taught elementary school for years and years. I remember meeting grown adults at her memorial service who were her students years ago. They had made their way back years later to pay their respects their favorite teacher. She was a dedicated wife and mother, stern but ever loving. She treated us grandkids like princes and princesses. When you sat on Grandma Coons' lap, you were the only thing that mattered in the world. She loved to play cards and board games, holidays, golfing with my Grandpa, and she adored her family. She was deeply wounded from the sudden and unexpected death of her nine-year-old son,

Doug, the uncle I never met. But she was a survivor, growing ever stronger, holding her family together, and giving of her love and joy and laughter to us all.

When she was diagnosed with breast cancer she fought like a prizefighter. She battled chemo, and she battled the cancer itself. I remember her losing her hair, and listening to her physical outcries of pain. She didn't know I heard because she refused to show it. She died just shy of her sixty-seventh birthday, and just before my sixteenth birthday in 1986. She is my hero, and I'm walking for her in the *Relay For Life* this weekend. I will carry her picture with me as I walk the survivor's lap on Saturday morning. And because of her, the gloves are off today.

I can't tell you how pissed I am at cancer today. I hate it, I hate it, I hate it. I hate it with a passion that I never have experienced before. This disease plays so dirty, so cheap, so foul. I hate what it does to people's bodies, to their minds, to their families, to their lives. And I want it to go away forever. I hate that it took my grandma from me when she and I were still young. I'm thankful I remember her as well as I do, but I grieve for my younger cousins and other people who got robbed of her beauty.

As I begin round three of chemo today I am remembering my Grandma and I'm choosing to move forward into this foggy week with her on my mind and heart. She is my reason for fighting this week. As for chemo itself, the staff almost didn't start it today because my white blood count was pretty low, right on the line. That explains why I started feeling lousy when I was fishing last Friday and on throughout the weekend. My body is taking a hit and is struggling to keep up with the treatments. I've lost 15 lbs. now, down to 190. I haven't seen that number in years. I'm wearing a size thirty-four in my jeans again! I wish it was because of something better like diet and exercise.

The nurse let me know that I really need to be careful to not get sick during this time. So again, if you are ill or have kids that are, please refrain from coming into contact with me. I can't afford to get sick. Thanks for again understanding my plight.

33 Born To Sing

April 23, 2009

I've been thinking a lot lately about the difference between "fate" and "destiny." Fate is something that renders us powerless. It's something that we cannot choose, for it chooses us. But destiny, well, that's something entirely different. I'm thankful for the difference because fate didn't choose this cancer, but I'm okay if destiny had it in store for me. Let me explain...

When destiny has something in store for us, there is a sense of empowerment that comes with it. We aren't thrown about to and fro by the waves it brings. No, in fact, I think destiny comes with a surfboard. It becomes a wave that we can choose to ride, even though there are moments that it feels like it is riding us. A few things have brought this whole topic to mind. The first is that my team, the *Army Of Love* for the upcoming *Relay for Life*, showed up at my doorstep today to take a photo. We wore the same matching team t-shirts and bonded over our common plight to end cancer. It was so reassuring to me to be surrounded by friends and family that are with me in this fight! The second is something the Apostle Paul wrote in his letter to the church he knew and love in Ephesus:

> For we are God's handiwork, created in
> Christ Jesus to do good works, which
> God prepared in advance for us to do.
> (Ephesians 2:10)

According to Paul, we are God's "handiwork," his genius, his beauty, his poetry, his works of art. And God has a plan for us, a destiny that we are asked to take it up daily. Like anything else from God, this is a gift that can lay unwrapped under the tree or can be opened and adored and put to use. The choice is ours.

What I've found, however, is that it isn't really a choice at all—at least not a very hard choice. When I was doing youth ministry, I would constantly mine rooms of kids to discover how God had gifted them. Sometimes, I admit, I had to look pretty hard. People, and especially teenage people, can be complete mysteries at first glance. But after mining a bit, each of them are amazingly gifted people and need us old folk to tell them the truth about who they are—amazing gifted people with purpose. But when I came across Heather, I didn't have to mine very deep to discover her gift. She could sing. And I don't mean just little. She could flat-out *sing*. God have given her pipes!

During a message one night at youth group, I was talking about how God had given each of us gifts. And I pointed at Heather and said, "Like Heather. Do you know what her gift is? What has God given her?" Everyone sitting around her mouthed the word *sing*.

"Exactly!" I said. "Heather was born to sing!" As those words left my mouth, I could visibly see Heather's love tank fill. She looked down, and grinned deeply. She blushed and, if I'm not mistaken, teared up a little. She knew her gift, and now others were noticing it! I knew it. Everyone around her knew it. *Heather was born to sing.*

Do people like Heather, people like you and me, have the choice to sing? Yes, but not really. I mean Heather could choose not to sing, but that would kill her. She was *born* to sing. But there was something inside her that *must* sing. So the choice was clear: *Sing.* She gave back her voice to the Giver of Voices and sang joyfully. She opened the gift and put it to good use. Use your gift! Shout if you have to! But don't miss out on the gift of God's destiny for you and for others!

Cancer is not my fate...but it is my destiny—a precarious gift that I have the choice to unwrap or leave unopened beneath the tree. I am choosing to unwrap it—as painful as that might be. But as I'm discovering, cancer has beautiful gifts to bear: Love, deep relationships with God and people, perspective, wisdom, patience, and many more life-lessons. I'm choosing to live this life to the full—it's the only life I have! And I'm living it even if it includes chemo, pain, questions, discomfort, fear, and disappointment...it is *my life.*

34 Life Is A Gift

April 27, 2009

One of the greatest Greek words is *zoe*. It means "life," but not just biological life like breathing and pooping. That kind of life is *bios*, where we get the word "biology." *Bios* is functional, earthly life. But *zoe* is a different kind of life. It's the kind of life that God gives. It's the kind of life that animates us, that beats deep within our souls, our hearts, our minds, and emotions. It's the life that God gives each of us that is beyond ordinary things like eyeballs, toenails, muscles, and colons. No, *zoe* is more profound. It is God-breathed, Spirit-infused, Jesus-given life. It's what makes our lives worth living.

Most often this kind of life is given to us by God through people. This past week I have been given *zoe-life*. It was given to me through the strength and love of my wife, Emily, and my kids and extended family. It was given to me through your prayers and encouragement via this *CarePage*. Zoe-life was given to me through several text messages of hope and love. It was given to me through my *Army of Love* who walked for twenty-four hours straight at the *Relay For Life* and raised over $5,000 for cancer research. It was given to me by my sister Cherie and her unexpected appearance at the *Relay for Life* Survivor Lap on Saturday morning. It was given to me through the memory and inspiration of my Grandma Coons as we walked in her honor around the track. It was given to me as my friend and brother and pastor Greg delivered what I consider to be the sermon of his life on Sunday. It was given to me in the warm greetings of those of you at church. *Zoe* was given to me through the care of my oncology nurses and their firm yet loving direction and concern for my health. It was given to me in the gift of fishing with close friends Tom and Ted, and of course, my Dad.

And finally, *zoe-life* was given to our whole family as we welcomed our newest family member, Zoe, our eight-week old, female, buff and white Cocker Spaniel! We chose the name Zoe because, right now, we need and welcome new, God-given life. She's awesome. She's darn cute. And yes, she's a lot of work!

Now, before I go any further, I want to address what I imagine is your concern: Why in the world would we introduce a puppy into the chaos we call our lives right now? Great question. (I'm beginning to ask it, too.) However, we have been talking about getting a dog for about two years. So this is not a spur-of-the-moment decision. We've weighed the consequences and have judged the good to outweigh the bad. And it truly does. What a wonderful distraction and infusion of life she is! Zoe has keyed in on my illness and knows when to jump up and cuddle with me when I'm down for the count in my chemo stupor. Other times she will keep pace with me as I shuffle about the house as I try to exercise my feeble body. It is becoming abundantly clear that as much as my family loves this dog, she is *my* dog. We have bonded over chemo. What a gift to have this furry little chemo partner. She is bringing me life in the midst of this craziness.

35 3 A.M.

April 30, 2009

Matchbox 20 sings a song called "3 A.M." I'm told that singer Rob Thomas wrote the song when he was a teenager and his mother was undergoing treatment for cancer. I imagine Thomas hearing his mother up in the middle of the night getting sick, feeling restless, and wanting it all to go away. The song vocalizes the feelings of this son of cancer: Awake, alone, scared, and overwhelmed by the power and evil of this disease.

Tonight I am that singer.

The cloudburst began at 3 A.M. last night and I couldn't, for the life of me, get back to sleep. I'm even taking the good sleeping pills! I think that my blood count is super low right now. Evidently, about nine days after chemo is the lowest of the blood counts. They call it the *nadir*, or low-point. It feels like someone has sucked all the energy out of me, like I've been sapped of all my strength and life. My limbs feel like cement, my heart is racing, and I can feel the anxiety rise in me like floodwaters. I'm spent. My voice is straining, my eyes are filled with tears, and I feel that I'm bottoming out. It's raining even though it's a bright, beautiful spring day.

This week has been a reality check. There are so many different realities to cancer, so many different levels that I'm experiencing. Just when I get through one, another one rears its ugly head and needs to be dealt with. It's like being caught in a torrent of waves breaking on shore. Just when one passes, another knocks me down again. The one I'm dealing with is the reality that my mind is way beyond my body. My mind tells me that I can do things like go fishing, exercise, and work, but my body is screaming, "NO!" And I get in over my head and physically bottom out.

This past Monday I almost blacked-out because I was trying to do too much when I was fishing. All I was doing was walking slowly around a small lake, but about halfway around the quarter-mile loop I sunk to my knees and had to call for help. Luckily I was around good friends who came to my aid, fed me energy bars and Gatorade. My oncology nurses were screaming at me in my head as I lay in the dirt and pine needles. They were telling me to stop trying to do so much and to give my body the rest that I need. I'm sure their yelling in my head will become a reality on Monday when I see them as I start chemo again. I just can't seem to understand that I'm not capable of doing all that I'm accustomed to in the past. It seems that I have cancer and therefore my body can't keep pace with my mental activity. I hate it!

I need wisdom and discipline to listen to my body and heed it. I'm realizing that I'm actually fighting for my life and I need to take the long-view and make short-term sacrifices for long-term gain. That's hard for me to remember!

But I also have hope, as the song says, "But outside it's stopped raining." I know one day, near or far, that the rain will stop. I hope it's sooner, to be frank. I'm tired of the rain. I have an inner-Seattle that is dank, dark and rainy. I'm dripping wet with no umbrella. Yet, in the middle of it all, I have hope. Though it wavers, my final hope is Jesus and his promises of his goodness and new life.

36 In The Darkest Of Moments

May 6, 2009

Today, I'll be honest, I feel like complete crud. I'm infusing chemo through this horrid little mechanical pump. It's like I have the worst flu ever, and it just keeps coming at me every time this little mechanical pump makes its little pumping noises. I can't help but hate it cycling that crap into me.

What a trip.

It makes me sick to my stomach each time I hear it. Luckily I get it out at 1:30 today and then the resting begins. I've been feeling better about two days after they disconnect me in the past, but it seems to last a little longer each round. Unfortunately, the effects are cumulative. So we'll just wait and see when I feel better after this round.

This Monday was supposed to be the beginning of my three-month sabbatical from ministry. I won a $15,000 grant to study Celtic Spirituality featuring a trip with our whole family to Scotland. Emily and I were going to spend a week on the Isle of Iona, the home of Celtic Spirituality. We were also going to do some other smaller trips, and spend three weeks at Lake Almanor just hanging out. Obviously that has changed. Fortunately, the Louisville Institute, the folks who awarded me the grant, have extended it to me for next year, so with God's grace, a year from now we'll get to take that sabbatical break.

One of the things that we were going to do each day was to practice the Celtic Spiritual tradition through morning and evening readings and prayers. Em and I decided that even though we're not doing sabbatical proper, that we would still begin this practice. As we read this morning, the reading invited us to be still and be aware of God's presence within and all around us (this is the big idea behind Celtic Spirituality as I understand it). I came to the reading with tears because I feel so lousy. It just upsets me to feel so sick. I hate it with a passion. I just want my body back! As I paused for the reading, listened and became aware of God's presence within me and around me, I heard God speak these gentle, graceful words:

James, I have not removed my hand from you. I am here in you and around you through your friends and family.

Wow. What amazing, beautiful words! God has been gracious to me and has come to me in the darkest of moments. He has been gentle, never harsh or angry, never judging or condemning. He has been always soft, loving, and full of grace. He reminded me that he is present, and thank goodness because my vision is limited to my discomfort and pain. Hearing his voice in prayer turned a dark, dreary, painful day into a day full of God's beauty, friendships, and possibilities, a totally different outlook: *Living rather than dying.*

37 A Begging Bowl

May 7, 2009

My body has been hijacked and I'm looking from the outside in at it. I still can't believe this is my life. It's not even that it's "happening to me," it's that it's happening at all. Who would have thunk it? I never would have thunk it! So strange, indeed. I was listening to U2's song "Moment of Surrender" and identified deeply with the words that speak of the singer's body becoming a "begging bowl," longing to get back to its original state, to being independent, to being whole again.

My body has truly become a begging bowl. It is begging for healing and normalcy, begging to be released from these dang chemo-toxins, begging to do what it is made to do. This body was made to cycle, walk, wrestle with my kids, dance, fly fish, and so much more. I long to be set free from cancer's grasp!

Two weeks ago when I about passed out from over-doing it while fishing, I sat on the porch putting my shoes on. As I messed with the knotted laces with my numb and toxic fingers, I had an honest conversation with God. I said, "God, you can have my life to do whatever you want. You know that. We made that deal a long time ago. All I have is yours. But, in the name of Jesus, I'm not done with this life yet! I'm not going down without a fight! *I AM SO NOT DONE, LORD.* I'm walking my girls down the aisle. I'm raising my boy as a man. I have great years of marriage and love to give to Emily. I have people to pastor. I have fish to catch! I AM SO NOT DONE!"

Giving up and throwing in the towel is not an option, though there are moments that it might seem the easier path. Living, all living—not just cancer living—requires courage. It takes courage to face the fullness of our lives—the fears, failures, embarrassments, resentments, doubts, and yes—cancers. I believe we each come to a point when we have to ask ourselves, "Will I claim this life as *my life*, or will I wish it away in the hope that it will be replaced with a charmed life, one free from pain, regrets, and failures?"

While I understand the urge to escape, I firmly believe in planting our feet on planet earth and engaging in the life God has given us. This is real time. This is real life. This is my life. Wishing it away isn't an option because I would miss out on the lessons and gifts this life has to give. However, that doesn't mean that I shouldn't fight through this life with courage, community, and prayer—they are our arsenals in the battles we face. To be sure, this life is a minefield of difficulties: Relationships failed, diseases caught, mistakes made. And every now and then we are certain to step on a few mines and receive the impact of the blow. We have the scars to prove it.

But I'll tell you this: I'd rather live with the scars than die a coward. That is the route I'm taking, that is the line I'm drawing.

38 A Sort Of Foot Wash

May 9, 2009

It is truly humbling to be on the receiving end of others' generosity in such truckloads. I believe one of the main reasons, if not the main reason, I have not felt abandoned by God in all of this is because I don't feel abandoned by the people of God. My community is the presence of God to me. It makes sense that the Body of Christ represents Christ in the world.

I had an experience a couple of weeks ago when I was fishing that tells this story. I was fishing into the evening on this little lake and it started to get cold. One of the main side effects of FOLFOX chemo is neuropathy which is code for "your hands and fingers hurt like hell." It was getting to the point where I couldn't really work my hands so I started paddling in on my little pontoon boat when all of a sudden BAM! My fly rod bent over and the fight was on! It was a nice eighteen-inch rainbow trout, a beautiful fish (and the only one of the night, by the way.) Okay, so that wasn't the point of my story, but it was worth re-living for a second...

The lesson came later on shore, on the deck of the little cabin we were staying in when I went to take off my boots. I simply couldn't do it. My fingers couldn't untie the laces and pry the wet boots off my numb feet. My hands hurt too much and simply were frozen. How helpless I felt! I couldn't untie my damn boots! I hung my head and just sat there in defeat. I was helpless. It was awful.

As I sat there dejected, my friend Ted saw my predicament. He asked if I needed help taking off my boots. "Yeah, that would be great. Thanks, man," I mumbled. It's strange, you know? I've led dozens of "foot washing" ceremonies in all my years of ministry, reenacting the night Jesus washed his disciples' feet in John 13, but I've never felt as humble in the act as I was in this moment. I realize it wasn't technically a foot washing, but it really was. The lack of feeling and strength rendered me powerless, and Ted did for me what I couldn't do for myself. Ted had to remove my boots or I was going to wear them and my waders for the rest of the evening. He understood my situation and was gracious, not making me feel awkward, but loved. As he untied my shoes, he gently retold a story of watching his junior high son washing the feet of a homeless person in San Francisco on a mission trip with his youth group. He recalled being so moved by the experience, and now I shared in the moment with him. All I could do is feel a great deep sense of gratitude.

That's how I feel now: Grateful. As people mow my lawn, come clean my house, feed us, and love my wife and kids, my feet are being washed. All I can do is say thank you.

39 Longing

May 20, 2009

Hoping daylight, watching sky,
Directionless looking,
Won't miss it.
Come good news,
Come trumpet-sound!
Shouts of joy, inquisitive faces,
Tears end,
Forever begins;
Ready now.

Please, wait.

Really?
Wait more?
Wait, watch, long, hope, expect, work, faith, look.
In-between is stuck,
Slow moments,
Slow tracking;
Choking smog, earthy dust, sad blood.

Levity comes like cool rain,
Returns to clouds.
So we wait,
Long,
Pray,
Love.

40 What More Could I Ask For?

May 24, 2009

Today I was reminded of the sufficiency of God. I was in church and it just re-occurred to me that life is precarious and that God is enough. A book I just finished confirmed this as well. It is a remarkable book called *Jesus Land* by Julia Scheeres, a memoir of her growing up in a conservative, abusive Christian home. It helped me refocus on God in a powerful way. I was reminded that for many people, God is brutal. The things that people and churches and ministries do in the name of God are sometimes disgusting. But when you find the real deal, when you come into the presence of the Living God, when you find that there is substance to it all and that substance is full of grace, truth, light, love, and life, it makes all the difference. God is no longer our enemy. He's our lover.

I found myself listening to our pastors differently today, through the ears and the heart of someone who has been abused by the church. I can report, gladly, that the "cringe factor" of Christianity was not present. I didn't feel put-off or rejected by God or God's people. Rather, I encountered a good God who is interested in my real life—cancer and all. I'm so thankful. I couldn't stand it if God were somehow angry with me and I was suffering because of something I did. Rather, I have the sense that God is shaking his head and crying with me, and standing with me in the uncertainty of it all. He's just here, and he loves me and that is why I can say that God is enough. What else could I ask for? A reason for cancer? I could be looking for that answer for a lifetime and still never know. But to know that God is with me is enough for me to move forward, to be present to others, and to give me a purpose and direction in life. What more can I ask for?

I'm two days away from round five. I can tell because I'm on edge. I get angry more easily, my skin a little thinner than usual. Just ask Emily. She'll tell you that I'm being a butt. Not that I need a defense, but chemo really does suck and I'd be lying if I said it was no big deal. It's a really big deal and I hate it with a freaking passion. I loathe the thought of being wiped-out again. But what's a guy to do? Get through it and move forward, knowing God is step-for-step by my side.

41 Not Alone

June 15, 2009

You can tell when I'm getting ready for another round of chemo because the updates start coming more frequently. I have had a great two weeks off. I've felt so good. I've spent a ton of time with my family, celebrating birthdays, taking my kids and wife on a number of dates, watching movies, keeping up with pro cycling in Europe, taking care of house projects, fishing (I think the old man out-fished me again), riding my stationary bike, going to church and celebrating our amazing God.

The highlight was watching thirty people get baptized in the creek behind the church. It was wonderful and also awful to watch all those baptisms. I wanted so badly to be down in the creek with my colleagues baptizing people with them. I felt truly sidelined and not part of God's will for me to not be using my gifts in that moment, though I was thrilled for those being baptized.

Oh, cancer affects me in so many unexpected ways! One moment things are just fine and the next I get smacked upside the head by something, a comment, or an event that I didn't see coming and think, "Oh yeah, I'm that guy," or, "Oh yeah, I *do* have cancer. I forgot!"

Just when I despaired, I read something that brought hope:

Why do you complain, Jacob?
Why do you say, Israel,
"My way is hidden from the LORD;
my cause is disregarded by my God?"
Do you not know?
Have you not heard?
The LORD is the everlasting God,
the Creator of the ends of the earth.
He will not grow tired or weary,
and his understanding no one can fathom.
He gives strength to the weary
and increases the power of the weak.
Even youths grow tired and weary,
and young men stumble and fall;
but those who hope in the LORD
will renew their strength.
They will soar on wings like eagles;
they will run and not grow weary,
they will walk and not be faint.

(Isaiah 40:27-31)

How I needed those words today, those promises! I am not alone! No, in fact, the One who made the heavens and earth is strengthening me. He understands, even though he didn't create my cancer, though somehow he allowed it to occur. He gets my life and offers his strength and courage to face it head-on, with courage and integrity. It gives me permission to not like my circumstances but face them anyway.

Wings like eagles...I want to fly!

42 Perspective

June 22, 2009

Well, I think the worst of round six of chemo is behind me. I'm still low and slow, taking it easy, trying not to overdo it, and rest. I'm so thankful for the time I have to simply *be* and not *do*. It allows me to focus on healing. I can't begin to imagine how so many people go through the rigors of chemo and then return to work a few days later. I feel truly grateful that I've been given this time to heal even as much as I hate not working because I love it so much. This is the *kiros*, God's exact right time, for me to be resting. It still doesn't add up entirely to me, but it is what it is and I'm riding the wave I've been given. It's either ride or get smashed into the sand, so I'm paddling out and looking for the set of waves that is to come.

Honestly, as I see the waves of round seven and eight coming, I can't imagine doing it again. But I trust that when those days come I'll be ready, or at the very least obedient, and go through with it. Pray that I keep my vigor and vitality, my will and desire to keep fighting and moving forward. My dad, who went through chemo last year, was right when he said that as you get further into chemo the will to fight weakens. I feel that already, and I'm potentially only halfway done.

How you view yourself and, more specifically, where you plant your feet, makes all the difference in the world when facing a rough time like this. I have realized that there is a zone that exists that is a "thin place," a space where heaven and earth seem to meet. My good friend and colleague, Greg Cootsona, describes what it was like for him to perform a wedding on the *Today Show* in 2006. He said that in the shadow of the New York skyline and in the face of doing a wedding on national TV, he felt scared. Who wouldn't? But then he described what I would call a "thin place" when his perspective switched. He realized that the message he had to offer in the wedding ceremony, the grace and love of God, was so much bigger than the New York skyscrapers and national TV that would soon broadcast him to millions of viewers. There is a certain power that comes from a realization like this. It's a magnanimous power, a power that doesn't come from within us, but a power that comes from elsewhere. There may have been seven million people watching the wedding on TV, but that pales in comparison to God's love. God's love is bigger than seven million people. Heck, God's love is bigger than a *google-flex* of people! (A *google-flex*, by the way, is the largest number in the world according to my children!) A realization like that can change any circumstance, including cancer.

The fuel that keeps me facing this disease and all these endless rounds of chemo is knowing that I belong, heart and soul, to God. God loves me and has bought me at the highest price: The life of his son. And that gives me power, a huge power, to keep going. I believe with all my being that God is bigger and more powerful than cancer will ever dream to be. Whether I live or whether I die, I have confidence that I am ultimately going to be healed.

Viewing my mortality in light of the hugeness of God is where God's timing, *kiros*, leads me to God's *shalom*, a peace and wholeness from God that transcends our circumstances. I am in the right place at the right time, doing what I need to be doing (*kiros*), though my task is the fight of my life. But dwarfing the skyscrapers of loss, pain, and suffering is God's presence and love—bigger than death itself! So I know, ultimately, that I'm going to be okay: *Shalom*.

Perspective changes everything. It's about remembering who you are, who you were created to be, and the power that exists beyond our limited creation. Having our feet planted in that soil—in that thin place—can help us face just about anything.

43 God With An Eye-Patch

June 28, 2009

The bad effects of treatment are decreasing as I get further away from my latest round of chemo. I just don't realize how bad I feel until I start feeling well. What a contrast! It's amazing what these drugs do to my body. Yet there continues to be good news in all of this. For example, I'm gaining weight, not losing it. And I still have not thrown-up except the day my surgeon told me that I would need to do chemo. The idea of chemo made me vomit, but the chemo itself hasn't. Whatever. I am counting my blessings.

I had the honor of reconnecting with some great friends today. As a friend and I were talking, we took stock of all the good that has come from my battle with cancer. It's only been a short four months since this began, but in that time I've met some amazing people, had some incredible conversations, been encouraged by so many, and have been met by God in some of the most gentle, loving, and peaceful ways. My faith has been built-up by this war, not torn-down. I have felt closer, not more distant from, God, my wife, my kids, my extended family, and my community. As sucky as the cancer and chemo are, they have brought many good gifts to me.

As my friend and I talked some more, we pondered the idea of predestination, the reformed Christian doctrine that God plans and conducts our lives in his sovereignty and wisdom. Entire churches and denominations are built around this doctrine. Indeed, lots of people base their faith on the doctrine, and it becomes very important for them to make sure it is water-tight, neatly wrapped with a bow, otherwise their faith comes unraveled. Though I'm a Presbyterian pastor and lover of John Calvin, I'm not too convinced of this doctrine he and his followers made famous—at least not right now. Predestination is a hurtful, abusive, crappy idea if it is used to forecast our lives and futures. In other words, I don't like the idea that God, in his sovereignty, planned for me to have cancer. That would be to say that *God planned for me to suffer*, that *God caused my suffering.* I can't go there! It makes God into a tyrant, a pirate. God with an eye-patch, hooked hand and a peg leg. Who wants to have a relationship with a tyrannical pirate-god? Not this pastor, not this cancer patient.

However, the doctrine of predestination is ever helpful when viewed in a rear-view mirror, in retrospect. As we look back on our lives, on our experiences, suffering, our "cancers," we begin to see how God was present, held us, strengthened us, and put the right people in our lives. He was provided for us. He was good, gentle, and peaceful—even if we didn't know it or feel it while in the middle of it. God didn't fail! Look back on your life and see if this isn't true. Has God disappointed you because he didn't meet your expectations, or has he been faithful in his loving presence? I'm betting on the latter. It's usually us that move away from God when things get tough. God promises to be with us in the thick of it:

> Never will I leave you; never will I forsake you. (Heb. 13:5)

As I look back on my life and all the crud I've gone through in relationships, disappointments, deaths, sickness, and now cancer, I can see how God has been present, worked, and brought beauty from the ashes called "my life." Did God plan for all that to happen? I honestly don't know. I have a really hard time believing that God plans for people to have cancer. Was I spared pain in all these difficult life circumstances? No. But can I believe that God is present and using this particular pain in my life to shape me, prepare me, teach me, and to help others? Absolutely.

44 *Domestiques*

July 6, 2009

Every July is a month-long celebration in the Coons house—it's *Tour de France* month. We are glued to the TV early in the morning watching this amazing race and the beautiful scenery of France. This year our house is decorated in yellow streamers and balloons, pictures of the cyclists, and our race pool charts. So far I'm in the lead in our pool, or as they say, I'm wearing the *maillot jaune*, or yellow jersey—the race leader's jersey. It feels good to be in the lead!

As great a distraction the *Tour de France* is, I'm keenly aware that I'll be starting round seven tomorrow. I just don't want to do chemo again! I hate the way it makes me feel and to know I'll be out of it for about two weeks just plain sucks.

I wish there was some way around this mountain, but there just isn't. I have to climb it. It reminds me of how cycling teams work together in the *Tour de France*. There is usually one guy who is the team leader, and everyone else on the team is called a *domestique*, or servant. That means they do the heavy pulls at the front of the *peloton*, or group of riders, to help their team leader make it over the mountains and through the flats, through vicious crosswinds, and down endless roads. They go get water bottles from their team cars and bring them back up the road for the leader. If a breakaway threatens their leader's lead, they go and chase down the threat and destroy the attempt at an upset. *Domestiques* will even give up their own bike to their leader if he crashes and his bike is damaged beyond riding condition. Racers like Lance Armstrong, Greg le Monde, and Eddy Merckx get all the glory for winning the *Tour de France*, but it is really their *domestiques* who do the most grueling work so their leader can cross the line in Paris first.

I need some *domestiques*. I need some helpers to pull me up the mountain and guide me through the valleys of round seven. Will you help again? I feel I go to that well often to draw from your deep faith, love and prayers each time I face another stage. So I'm asking again. Pray, pray, pray. Pray that I have the very strength of the resurrection to carry me through this round. Pray I'll sleep and that God meets me in the pain. I believe he has, does, and will, but I want you to remind him. I can't help but think that God is on the hook for this one. When he told the Israelites that, "I will be your God, you will be my people," (Genesis 17) he made a deal with us, *with me*. Please ask God to see through his deal with me this week.

My sister, Cherie, will join me for my infusion tomorrow. In a strange way I'm excited for her to join me in my world. One of the most powerful messages of love that I've received throughout this journey is the willingness of different people, like Cherie, to just show up and join me. In fact, the times I have felt most loved are when people simply come alongside our family and simply hang with us. I have found this so much more helpful that when people say, "If there's anything I can do, let me know." I can't come up with ways for people to help, especially when I feel like crud. It takes too much energy to invent helpful tasks for people to do. But when people take initiative and show up, even if I'm not up for a visitor, it means the world to me. When people just drop off groceries, come and do our dishes and laundry unannounced, or help with the kids, it communicates their willingness and love for us in a down-to-earth, I'm-not-afraid-of-rolling-up-my-sleeves-and-getting-dirty kind of love. Use your creativity in loving others! Take initiative! It's no surprise that God loves us this way in that he comes to us first. He doesn't ask, "How can I help you?" He just helps in creative, life-giving ways. So go for it!

45 Keeping It Real

July 11, 2009

Up till this point I've felt that I've been standing out in a rushing river fighting my best against the current. And thus far I feel that I've put up a pretty good fight. I do a lot of fishing in streams and rivers, and I know how to navigate them pretty well. I know how to avoid falling in or getting swept away. Likewise, I've been around suffering and cancer enough in my life that I've felt pretty secure in facing this challenge, staying strong, not getting swept away.

It changed this week. Sure, I've done six other rounds of chemo, but the game changed this week. In fact, it ain't no game at all. Round seven took me down in about two seconds and swept me away. I've never faced something so challenging in my life. I truly feel that I'm putting my life on the line to fight through this. The river swept me away this week and I'm being taken downstream against my will. I can't fight it any longer. I thought I was at the end of my rope before...I guess I had some more length to go, because I now feel that I can't go any lower.

I'm done.

Today, as I was on the massage table, I was thinking about how people who have had cancer call themselves "survivors." If and when I get through this, I will proudly call myself a "survivor:" That is exactly what I will have done—survived. That is about all I can imagine doing right now. Being productive and lively are the furthest things from my mind. It's all I can do to breathe in and out.

Sorry to drone on about how rough it is right now. I don't know what else to do except open up and let others know what's going on in the hope that God might meet my family and surprise us and make things a little easier. I won't speak for the rest of my family, but I know I could use a fresh outpouring of God's presence and grace. I feel that I've been running around with a bucket trying to catch drops of God when what I really need is the torrential outpouring of his presence. I'm worn out from trying to chase God around. I'm ready to be found again.

Just keepin' it real…

46 Words

Words are powerful. They have the ability to make one feel as good as can be, or they can make one feel awful. Fortunately, the words of my *Army of Love* have made me feel great. In fact, their words have made me feel the very presence of God who journeys with me through this long, dry desert.

Unfortunately, though, occasionally someone trys to placate me with cheap words. As I talked with a dear friend on the phone today, I commented that I've become bitter and jaded by this last week of chemo-suffering. When my unfortunate friend attempted to identify or relate to my suffering, his words fell short, making me feel small and unheard. I was probably a little quick to dismiss his attempt to love me, turning into a sixteen-year-old version of myself and silently cussed him out in my head. I wanted to scream, "You don't know me! You don't know my suffering! Nobody knows my suffering!" Fortunately, I quickly realized that I'm almost forty and that kind of behavior doesn't get one far in life, nor does it solve the current problem.

So, to those who have said things like, "I don't have the magic words to make it go away," or, "We're still here and praying for you," thank you for your presence and love. Those are the perfect words. They don't assume to know how I'm feeling, but they communicate your presence, attention, and love. Perfect. Keep it coming! They are words of life to me.

47 Affirming Life

July 13, 2009

I feel that I turned a corner last night and today I'm starting to recover. I'm not out of the woods yet. I still have a lot of digestive problems, fatigue, mouth sores, hair loss, and nausea. But I'm a lot better off than I was even a day ago. It has taken me longer to recover in these later rounds. I realize how easy the first five rounds were, though I wouldn't have said so at the time. Those rounds were kid's play, I tell you. I'm into the big leagues now, or so I think. I can't imagine what others go through.

I talked with a woman in the doctor's office the other day and she said she's been receiving treatments since January and is scheduled to end in December. That's serious. But I've found with suffering it doesn't really do to compare. Suffering is just suffering. Every person's journey and pain are different and unique to them. I'm just sorry there has to be a journey that involves suffering at all.

So for today, I am choosing to affirm life. I am choosing to appreciate my family, my dog, a freshly cleaned house, plans to have lunch with my friend Bill tomorrow, the *Harry Potter* book I just started, the doorknob I fixed in the laundry room, my friend Mark at the bike shop who showed me the new carbon-fiber bikes just in, the *Tour de France* and Lance Armstrong, cool air conditioning on a hot summer day, my friend who wants to come visit me, another friend from out of town who is here in Chico and will visit this week, the anticipation of getting away with Emily next week to Sonoma to celebrate her fortieth birthday, ice cream, and beer. That's the list I can come up with for now. Let's affirm life together.

48 The Silence Of God

July 19, 2009

While I was down and out a week or so ago, I realized something that I hadn't felt in years: *The silence of God.* It was freaky. Usually, when I cry out to God, I find him readily present. But whether it was the darkness of my valley and depression or the numbness of my senses from chemo, I couldn't hear or sense God anywhere. He was lost to me, nowhere to be found. He could have been shouting his love at me and I could have just missed it. Or, more than likely, it is just plain hard to hear or sense God when you're suffering. It was unlike anything I've experienced before. He still seems distant, to be honest.

It brings up that whole problem of pain and suffering: Why does God promise good for his children and then allow them to suffer? I don't get it. What could possibly be the point of it all? To teach us some lesson? To build our character? To test our will? Probably. And those are ultimately great things when we get *there*, but what about *here*? What about *now*? Why are we allowed to suffer here and now? I don't know. I wish I had a better answer, but I don't. I'm stumped.

I may not have an answer to why we suffer, but I do know this: *We will suffer.* It is a universal truth that we cannot escape. But rather than get stymied by suffering, we can choose to move with suffering as it ebbs and flows rather than ignore or resist it.

I choose, therefore, to invite and allow others to stand in the gap between God and me during this time of silence-suffering. I imagine flipping suffering off when I let others into my pain and ask them to pray for and encourage me. As I write transparently about my hurt, loneliness, grief, and pain, I am drawing that ever so important line in the sand, dividing myself from the circumstances that dog me. It is the way I remind myself that I am not my suffering. I am much more what this moment in my life would have me believe.

49 Obstacles into Opportunities

August 4, 2009

Why do the words *right* and *hard* go hand-in-hand? It's the *right* thing for me to complete all twelve rounds of chemo. But to do so will be *hard*. Why can't the *right* thing be *easy*, or at least a little *less hard*? I guess that is just the way cancer rolls. It makes life *hard* on its victims. I hate this disease.

It took me four weeks between rounds of chemo to get to number eight, which I am currently infusing now. After this week, I have four more rounds, and with an average of three to four weeks off between rounds, you do the math. When we started treatments, we thought we'd be done in August. I anticipated being back to work and in the full swing of life by mid-fall. It's not looking that way now.

This cancer journey is full of the unexpected, trials, tests, and obstacles. Lately I've been re-reading Lance Armstrong's autobiography, *It's Not About the Bike*. What a tenacious S.O.B.! That guy is remarkable in his accomplishments, but even more remarkable is the fabric of his humanity. As with all of us, who we are is greatly determined by the first few years of our lives when we learn what it is to be human. This was the case with Armstrong as well. He had a tumultuous youth, though he doesn't report it as such. He made it sound normal, but it was strained. His mother was married and divorced several times, and for the most part, Armstrong didn't have a steady male role model in his life. However, he had a remarkable mom who would tell him from a very young age, "Make an obstacle an opportunity, make a negative a positive."[1]

Lance learned that lesson, didn't he? He's turned what was certainly a death sentence into a global campaign to stamp out cancer. He turned his pain of chemo and surgery into learning how to be patient with suffering. He learned how to endure pain on a bike over long periods of time, going really fast, and winning the *Tour de France* seven times and came close to winning again this year after a four-year break from the sport.[2]

But Lance is just another person, too. He is a normal man who took what he learned in his suffering and turned it into opportunities for success and victory. That is something every human can learn to do. It's not about the bike; it's about the human spirit. It's about letting God into your journey and allowing him to heal, love, guide, strengthen, and walk with you. And the best way I've learned to allow God in is to let others in, letting them know the depths of what is going on and allowing them to support, encourage, and love you. They become God's voice and presence during suffering. It starts with a choice to turn our obstacles into opportunities for growth, strength, and victory.

My journey has taken so many twists and turns. Unexpected obstacles have landed in our path. If you saw my scars as I do each day, you would be reminded of the pain that I've been through. My hands and feet are constantly burning from the inside out, numb from the *Oxolyplatin*, a condition called *neuropathy*. I've lost a ton of muscle and strength. Each day as I wake up I look at all the hair on my pillow that once was part of my head. I take a load of pills each day, have to drink a million gallons of water per day to stay hydrated, and consider myself a human pin-cushion for all the shots and blood draws I receive. I have to constantly battle my mind, determining that I'm not going to die from this disease. Sometimes I lose the mental battle, but sometimes I win—it just depends on the day. I have learned the language of cancer, become an armchair oncologist, and met some of the most remarkable people who are fighting this disease. My full-time job is to beat cancer and make it through this season with my life and family intact. This is a huge obstacle in my path.

But it is also a huge, golden, amazing opportunity. It's an opportunity to have God re-define my circumstances and his love for me. Allen, one of the pastors at our church, in a message on Psalm 23, talked about that line that says, "Though I walk through the valley of the darkest shadow, you are with me. Your rod and staff, they comfort me." He went on to share a personal story of a dark shadow valley he once walked through, and how God met him and guided him through it. This spoke the loudest to me because I've struggled feeling abandoned by God in the midst of my fight with cancer.

He also talked about scars, literal scars on our bodies as well as scars in our hearts, minds, and souls from life's hardships and suffering. He offered this perspective, "Maybe our scars aren't evidence of God's abandonment of us. Maybe they are signs of God not being through with us yet." Isn't that refreshing? I have massive scars on my body because God isn't through with me yet. They aren't signs of God abandoning me at all! They are signs that God is saving me! I go through awful, body-racking therapies not because God is absent, but because God is present and offering me new life. I'm losing my hair not because God has forgotten me, but because he has remembered me, loves me, and isn't through with me yet. This is my chance to be born all over again, to become a new person shaped, but not defined, by the suffering of cancer. What an opportunity! What a gift! It is with that new perspective that I face round eight of chemo this week.

50 Natural, Neutral, Evil

August 6, 2009

I continue to marvel at how life just isn't fair. And that would be okay if I wasn't brought up in a culture that told me that it should be. Sometimes stuff just happens and there is no rhyme or reason for it. It just is. So much of what happens to us or around us is natural, like death, or neutral like getting sick, or evil, like war. Our character is proven by how we respond to these natural, neutral, or evil circumstances. How we respond to life's injustices, illnesses, and trials says more about who we are than the fact that we go through them. Patience is the key. Not reacting too quickly is crucial. Keeping focused, perspective, and our cool is absolutely essential. So much is out of our control, but what we can control is our reaction to the stuff of life.

One of my most often uttered prayers is for wisdom so I can make my way through all the stress and strains that life serves us. "God, give me wisdom on how to respond! Help me respond as you would. Help me reflect your grace, your truth, and your life as I move throughout this world and all it has to dish-out. Keep me above reproach and petty even-making. May my response to what I consider life's injustices reflect your Kingdom and bring you glory, because at the end of the day, I recognize that it's not about me—it's about you and the life and hope you bring. So let me resolve to be about that, not about me."

All right, I think I've talked myself off the ledge for now.

51 The Rest Of My Life

August 11, 2009

If ever there was a time to get cancer, now is the time. There has been no greater time in history to get it. The advances they are making in cancer research and treatments are staggering. If I had been diagnosed with stage three colon cancer twenty years ago it would be a death sentence. But as it is now, I have really great chances of surviving and never dealing with cancer again. That's a miracle in itself. So while I'm cursing the drugs they give me, I also recognize their amazing value and significance, not just for me, but for so many others as well.

I'm doing pretty well this week. I've been tired and still feel (and taste) the chemo and *Neulasta*, a drug that increases the production of white blood cells. I've been able to take walks, get on the bike trainer and sweat it up, and be with my friends and family on my terms. Emily said I did much better this round than round seven. I bounced back quicker than I remember, but honestly all the rounds have kind of melded together in my fuzzy mind. I can't keep track of the day of the week much less my recoveries from chemo. Everything is kind of blurry right now.

For whatever reason (God), I've been coming across several books and articles about survivorship. So much of what is written and taught about cancer has to do with the diagnosis and treatment stages. No doubt, those have been helpful. But as I am approaching the back nine of chemo treatments I'm starting to think about survivorship. I don't want to make the leap too soon, but I feel that God is beginning to prepare me for the next leg of this journey. What has dawned on me that living with cancer, even if I don't actively have it, is something that will be with me the rest of my life. From what I've read and heard, the disease doesn't leave you alone once you're told that you don't have it any more. For example, my doc let fly that I would be having yearly PET/CT scans once I'm done with chemo. Wow! Those are stressful tests because they reveal so much. I can't imagine being several years down the road and getting a scan, then waiting for the results, reliving all the fear and memories of the past few months. Can you imagine the nightmare that will be, waiting to hear if it has come back or not? Blah!

All that being said, I'm taking it as a good sign that I am being prepared for the next stage of this journey. I'm certainly ready for this current one to be done, so flip that page!

52 A Collision

August 14, 2009

The past few days have been a collision of the highest of highs with the lowest of lows. The highs: Watching the Giants vs. Dodgers game, seeing the Giants pull out a win in the tenth with a walk-off home-run, spending a great day with my dad and Jake at the ball park, watching Jake get the game for the first time, getting autographs, hot-dogs, and soda. Another high: A great visit from our dear friends from Santa Cruz. What a great reunion for us! Also, realizing again that I have the most amazing woman for a wife. I couldn't live without her. She is my life-blood. Finally, I have an incredible God who has been answering my prayers, showing up through friends and loved ones, reminding me that I'm not alone. God is here fighting for me. My list goes on…

The lows: I've been experiencing fear like I've never known before. I've been having panic attacks that paralyze me and cause strange out-of-body sensations that the nurses have helped me understand as chemo side effects. I've also been experiencing deep, deep fatigue. Each time I think I've reached the end of my rope, I find that there is a little bit more length, lowering me deeper and deeper into the pit of misery. When does this rope end?

Please pray for me. I've said this before, but this time I say it with a new urgency: I am riding your coattails because I have nothing left in my tank. I am exhausted like I've never been before. Empty. Game over. As close to death as I've ever felt. Ka-put. Done. *Finito.* Game over. I'm scared. I'm tired. I'm afraid. I'm weak. I'm finished.

Yet I have hope and want to keep fighting, but I just can't seem to find the reserves to keep going. So I need you.

53 Hope Deferred

August 22, 2009

I love new days. New days bring new perspectives, new possibilities, and new hope. Most mornings I sit in our backyard and enjoy the garden, the fresh, cool air, and take in the newness that comes in the dawn. Lately, I've been drawn to our morning glories that are crawling their way up our fence. They have the most amazing magenta flowers that come out in the early part of the day, but in the afternoon and evening they close back down—kind of like me. I seem to do great in the mornings, but by mid-afternoon and evening I close back down again. I don't have much energy after the sun goes down. I find myself shuffling around like an old man, gasping for breath, and winded at the top of the stairs. A walk around the block is like a marathon. Fortunately, I usually have my dog Zoe on a leash and she manages to pull me around and keeps me moving.

But I love mornings the most. They remind me that there is still hope. I'm clinging to hope these days. I just finished round nine of chemo. In a conversation with one of my nurses yesterday I asked if she had ever seen someone go beyond eight rounds of FOLFOX. She said no, she hasn't. Everyone stops at eight, she said. Nobody she has seen has made it beyond. She's been doing this for close to twenty years, too. Amazing. The caveat is that most the people taking FOLFOX are twice my age. I'm positive that being under forty is to my advantage—I'm young and strong! Plus, I only have to suck down three more rounds of chemo. I'm feeling hopeful and can see the light at the end of the tunnel. However, I know it will be a rough road between here and there.

The neuropathy in my hands and feet hit an all-time new level of pain this round. I can't believe that twenty million Americans live with this condition, mostly from diabetes. My neuropathy is due to the exposure I've had to the toxins in chemo. It feels like my hands are on fire from the inside out. The trick with toxin-caused neuropathy is to endure the pain so the chemo can kill the cancer without inflicting permanent nerve damage to my hands and feet. I'm the only one who knows the pain and its effects, so it's my call to say when enough is enough. I hesitate to take drugs to mask the pain because the pain is my only metric of how my nerves feel. There is a fine balance between killing cancer and killing my nerves. It is temporary suffering for long-term gain.

My problem, however, is that I'm used to instant gratification and quick solutions to my problems: "Here, take this pill and you'll feel better!" Or, "You don't have to wait to buy that, you can use CREDIT!" You know the story. Well, cancer treatment is the exact opposite of that story. Chemo is a series of painful deposits in an account of suffering for living life later. Why is it that all the most meaningful commitments in our lives (marriage, parenting, integrity, getting treated for disease) require patience, the long-view, perseverance, relying on hope, waiting, long-term investments, and faith? Why couldn't we just get what we want now? Cancer flies in the face of our Western instant gratification mores. This disease will have none of our American culture. It eats it for lunch and makes us much more Eastern in our approach to life. *Wait. Patience. Invest. Learn. Breathe.*

I'm learning the lesson of hope deferred while I'm clinging to the foretastes of that hope that come each morning, trusting that a whole new day is awaiting me and my family…a day without cancer.

54 Talking Or Acting

August 29, 2009

I've had a pretty good week health-wise, although I've been really tired the last couple of days. My fatigue level goes up and down like a yo-yo. Chemo is so damn unpredictable. My blood counts came back and they are good! I'll start round ten on Monday. Double-digits! I can't believe I'm making it towards the end. I was so set on making it to round eight for so long that it seems miraculous to make it this far. If my counts remain good between rounds I'm due to finish round twelve the first week of October. I can almost taste the finish line from here.

This week I started a new medication that has a dual purpose. One purpose is to help ease the pain of my neuropathy, which I'm really grateful for because it hurts like hell. I have numbness and burning in my hands all the time now. The second purpose of the med is an anti-depressant. I met with my doc the other day and we determined that I'm battling depression in the midst of all this stuff happening in my life. Not surprising. He assured me that it is totally normal—and expected—that battling for your life will lead to anxiety attacks and depression. Check. That's me. That's my life.

I tell you this so you know how to pray, but also to let you know that keeping depression and anxiety to yourself doesn't lead to health. Silence leads only to feeling more isolated and alone and deepens the depression.

As we experience loss, fear, sadness, frustration or any other negative feeling, we are faced with a choice: *Talk* it out or *act* it out. I've battled depression in the past, and I've learned that putting our feelings and emotions into words is the key to walking through those dark times. It forces us to become aware of our feelings and explore them more accurately. It also disarms the fear and anxiety we have about our feelings as we share the burden of them with our friends and families. Often our feelings are too much for us to handle alone. We are dwarfed by some of the circumstances of our lives— things like cancer, a death of a loved one, a loss of a job or a divorce can make us feel small and helpless. The pain of living can become too much to bear on our own. Therefore, talking out our feelings and emotions and getting the appropriate help from friends, or even trained people and/or medications, leads to our health and freedom.

The alternative is to suffer in silence, to allow our fears, frustrations, and feelings to become our jailers, locking us up in the cycle of pain that comes with loss and hurt. Once we start down this lonely road, what we don't realize is that the emotions and feelings need to get out, and in fact will be released one way or the other. Like containers under pressure, those feelings will leak out, and left untended, take the form of despair, panic, anger, rage, abuse, blame, violence, self-mutilation and even suicide. As my good friend Brian Morgan says, "Those feelings that we don't talk out, we act out."

Please say a prayer for me as I work through the darkness of my circumstances and slowly move toward God's light and life once again. I'm confident, with the help and support I have, that I will make it there yet again. Just another journey I get to take.

55 A Declaration

September 6, 2009

This past week has been the worst so far. It seems that each round gets tougher. As I've been battling and waiting the chemo out, I was thinking about the things that are truest about me:

❖ I declare that I am not cancer; I am Jim Coons.

❖ Cancer doesn't get to define me even though it wants to.

❖ I declare my life is hidden with Christ in God—a place that cancer can never touch.

❖ I declare that I hate cancer because it forces me to be selfish. I do not like being selfish.

❖ I declare that I'm going all twelve rounds of chemo. Not just for me, but for Emily, Julia, Jakob, and Eliza Kate. They are keeping me in the game.

❖ I declare that each day I will defy cancer by walking, riding my bike, or seeking some form of movement.

❖ I declare that I won't let cancer beat me.

❖ I declare that my plans are always going to be subject to change, but I'm learning to be okay with that new reality.

❖ I declare that I will work actively to be transparent about who I am, how I feel, and my needs to my community.

❖ I declare that I will always make an effort to look up, laugh, love, and live.

56 Waiting

September 18, 2009

I don't wait well. And in the world of cancer there is a lot of waiting. I mean A LOT of waiting:

Wait for tests to come back.

Wait for appointments.

Wait for blood counts to rise.

Wait.

Wait.

Wait.

I hate waiting! I just learned that my blood counts haven't gone up again. That means I'll have another blood draw on Sunday to see if the count goes up over the weekend. If not I'll have to endure yet another week waiting for the next round.

We're so close to being done and each delay pushes the finish line that much further away. I just want this to be over. What I really feel is frustrated that my body isn't recovering the way it did. Chemo suffering is not vanishing; it's just waiting in the wings, waiting to take center stage again in this unfolding cancer drama.

Right on cue, just as I was feeling frustrated with all this waiting, God interrupted my pity party with his opinion on the subject of waiting. How often does this happen in our lives, that God has a different perspective on our human circumstances? All too often. As I was reading Psalm 27 this morning, I read this:

> I remain confident of this:
> I will see the goodness of the
> LORD
> in the land of the living.
> Wait for the LORD;
> be strong and take heart
> and wait for the LORD.
>
> (Psalm 27:13-14)

I am faced with a choice again: To be discouraged by all this waiting, or to wait for the Lord in the midst of waiting for my blood counts to go up. I am more convinced than ever that God is good and working on my behalf, bringing about healing and wholeness to my body and soul.

And my job? To wait for the work to be accomplished. And your job? To pray for my patience as well as allow the lesson I'm learning teach you so you can face your own times of discouragement, to wait and trust that God is really up to something, even if you can't see it or feel it.

57 The Next Chapter

October 4, 2009

Tomorrow is round twelve—the last round of chemo. It has been a long journey to get to this point. Round twelve, wow! I had my doubts that I'd make it all the way through. I'm trying to be excited, too, but going through chemo again will be tough. I think I'll save my excitement for the end of this week.

As I am quickly approaching the end of this chapter, I am also trying to prepare for the next. It's a mind-bender to get my head around the fact that I'll be done with weekly (almost daily) doctor visits, blood tests, and being poked and prodded. Just like that, *snap*, it's going to end. I'll have follow up appointments and tests, but nowhere near the pace of the last eight months. It has been my full-time job to fight cancer, and now I feel I'm being kicked to the curb. I'm nervous about this because I've grown accustomed to being around doctors and nurses, being able to ask my questions and feel their regular support. What if something happens and need their immediate attention? What happens if something goes wrong and I have to *wait* for help (have I mentioned I hate waiting)? I'm used to their instant touch, their instant drug-fixes, and their instant assurance.

On the other hand, I'm looking forward to simply resting and not having the pressing anxiety of more chemo. I'm looking forward to the next chapter, working out, biking on real roads, and not feeling constantly chemicalized. I'm looking forward to regaining the feeling in my hands and feet, not dealing with mouth-sores, nausea, and constant fatigue. I get to play with my kids again without restraint and I get to go back to work without reservation! I get my life back!

The biggest challenge I face, though, will be to get my head around what I've just been through. What is the meaning of the last eight months? What life lessons has this taught me? How will this experience affect my ministry? How am I different because of cancer and chemo? What has this taught me about the kind of husband and father I want to be? About the kind of friend I want to be? I don't have the answers at this point, but I'll be seeking them over the next several months and years—maybe for a lifetime. A person can't go through what I've just been through and walk away unchanged. I know I've changed, but I just don't know how and to what extent.

And so it is, with great excitement and awareness of the upcoming chapter that I head into this final chemo week. As always, I appreciate your prayers and messages.

58 Riding Into Paris

October 7, 2009

In the midst of my chemo fog I am rejoicing this morning. I will be disconnected from the last of my chemotherapy at 11:30 today. It's hard to believe that it is coming to an end. It doesn't seem real. I am imagining myself as a *Tour de France* rider pedaling his way into Paris onto the cobblestone streets of the *Champs-Élysées*, taking those final turns and striving for the finish line. I'm looking back on all the mountains and valleys I've come through, the exhilarating downhills and grueling mountain passes. I'm thankful for all the *domestiques*, those who have pulled me up the hills and guided me through the treacherous stretches with their presence, prayers, and encouragements. It has not been easy. No, in fact it has been the hardest challenge of my life. It has tested and tried every fiber of my being. I've been brought to the very edge physically. I've been over the edge mentally. And I've been stretched more spiritually that I have ever been.

They say that once a cyclist rides the *Tour de France*, three straight weeks on a bike, over two thousand miles of riding, that his body is forever changed. His muscles and metabolism are permanently different. His mind is permanently changed. I can see how, after facing so many grueling moments along the way, a rider would look at mountains and valleys differently. What seemed like challenges before probably seem insignificant distractions now. What seemed like impossibilities in the former life seem totally possible—almost easy—compared to the challenges faced in *le Tour*. This cancer race has had the same effects on me. I am a changed man. I've tolerated more physically than I ever thought possible. I've weathered more mentally than I ever. I've been to the brink of sanity, stared death in the eye, and walked away. And I've gone rounds with God, blow for blow, question after unanswerable question. I can't help but feel like Jacob, having wrestled with God and refused to let him go without his blessing (Genesis 32). I'm not the same man I was a year ago. What an amazing journey this has been.

I plan to keep posting updates, keeping you informed on my recovery. But let's pause and give thanks to God for getting us to Paris.

59 It's Not Fair!

October 14, 2009

How many times in our lives do we utter the words, "It's not fair!" Probably more than we realize. We Americans prize fairness. We're taught that things need to be equal at an early age. We learn it in sports: If the other team scores a goal, we have to score a goal. We learn it at Christmas as children: "She got six presents and I only got five!" We learn it as teenagers: "I want to be as good-looking as her." We continue on as adults: "I want the same raise that he got!" Or, "The neighbors got a new boat, we should get one, too!" Fairness is so subtle that often we don't realize we're caught up in it. It's part of the air we breathe in North America. Fairness is a right, right? And our competitive spirits ensure that it remains so.

Yesterday Emily and I were eating lunch and talking about fairness. I remarked that it's a good thing that God doesn't operate on the basis of fair; otherwise Emily would get cancer, too! Think about that for a second. If fairness is our right, something owed to us by the universe, then it has to apply to pain and suffering just as it does to Christmas presents and boats. Fairness, at its core, has to be *fair*. Both sides of human existence have to live under the fairness principle, the good side and the bad side.

I'm sure glad God doesn't live under the fairness principle. We're reminded that he doesn't operate this way when Jesus told the story of the workers in the vineyard. Some of the workers were paid a full day's wage for working only a short time. Of course, those who had really worked a full day and were paid the same as the so-called slackers, were enraged. They complained that it wasn't fair, that they should get paid more than those who only worked the last hour of the day. Then the vineyard owner set them straight. He reminded them that it was his vineyard and his money. He paid what he thought was fair. He had agreed on a wage with them already. He paid them that wage. Then he asked the real question:

> Are you envious because I'm generous?
> (Matt 20:15)

Thank God he doesn't play by our rules. If he did, we would short-circuit his generosity. I'm so thankful that life isn't fair. I don't want to see Emily get cancer. I don't want my suffering to be equalized. I want it to be unfair so God gets to remain generous. The other option turns God into a tyrant, always keeping score, always making sure that everyone is happy, or at least equal. The last time I checked, however, life isn't about being happy or equal. It's about God and his generosity, his love, his grace, and his life that he wants to give us, free of charge regardless of whether we deserve it or not. Thank God he's not fair!

60 Disneyland And U2

October 27, 2009

We just got home from our homemade make-a-wish trip to Southern California where we went to Disneyland and saw a U2 concert at the Rose Bowl in Pasadena. We had such a great time!

Disneyland was incredible! It truly transported us into a magical kingdom where roller coasters, princesses, and swimming pools reigned. We arrived at the *Disney's Grand Californian Hotel*, an amazing turn-of the century themed Californian lodge complete with redwood trees, grand ballrooms, and sounds of birds and wild animals pumped through their state-of-the-art invisible sound system. We were so excited to arrive that I forgot to park the car! I just left it in front of the hotel where the valet and bellboys helped us unload and we ran straight for our room, swimming pool, and Downtown Disney. It wasn't until after dinner about six hours later that I remembered that I had left the car parked in front of the hotel, doors and windows wide open, keys still in the ignition. Tell me I wasn't ready for vacation! Fortunately the hotel wasn't as absent-minded as me and parked it for us.

Shortly after arriving in our rooms, a bellboy came to our door and delivered two or three giant plastic tubs and coolers filled with snacks, chips, fresh fruit, and canned drinks: All the essentials for theme-park lunches. I had no idea who had sent this amazing gift, so I called the lobby and inquired. It turned out that one of my longtime closest friends and former sixth grade pen pal from Long Beach had been following my *CarePage* and knew we were headed to Disneyland to rest and celebrate the end of treatment. She and her family not only provided these gifts, but also paid for our hotel bill! Wow! When I told our family about the gift, we all jumped up and down on our hotel beds, then instantly jumped in the hotel pool and ordered fancy drinks with little umbrellas. What a gift! We felt completely removed from the cancer saga we've been through. We kept looking at one another in amazement and relief. We were on the other side of chemo! Finally! What a huge relief!

As if Disneyland weren't enough, we then drove to Pasadena to see U2 in concert at the Rose Bowl! As we drove up to Pasadena where we had lived for four years during seminary, we were able to show our son Jakob the hospital where he was born. It was awesome to see him connect his birth with the life he now lives. He seemed proud and excited to learn about that part of his story.

Anticipation rose as the day went on, closer to moment we had been awaiting for months—the concert. U2 would be playing live with the Black Eyed Peas at the Rose Bowl. And what a show it was! The kids loved it, though Jakob fell dead asleep in my lap about halfway into the U2 show. I caught glimpses of the concert on the video screen through the standing crowd in front of me while my boy slept. Eventually we needed to leave the concert because he was so done and so tired (as was his dad!). I am admittedly sorry that I didn't get to see the whole concert, however I am a dad before I am a U2 fan. I only get to be a dad once, but there will be lots of other concerts.

Our amazing trip came to an abrupt halt as I came home to have my PET/CT scan to determine whether or not I have any sign of disease. I'll get the results in a few days. More waiting…

Laying on the table, being injected with nuclear isotopes, hearing that machine whirr and whirl around me, and now waiting for the results from the "table of truth" has been a rough way to re-enter reality. "Oh yeah, I'm battling cancer here," I'm reminded. It reminded me of the space shuttle reentering the earth's atmosphere: Red-hot, stressed, no communication, blacked-out, and landing a little wobbly.   We had a wonderful time forgetting all about cancer at Disneyland and U2, but now cancer is being shoved back in our face with its ever-present threat and pain. Of course I'm anxious about the results, though I'm optimistic. I can't imagine that I have any cancer left in my body after all the chemo I've received. It would be unimaginable.

61 Welcome Ned!

October 29, 2009

They are the words that every cancer patient longs to hear: "No Evidence of Disease" or NED. It is why we hang in there for so long, endure such grueling treatments, undergo so many tests, and allow surgeons to cut us open time and again. It's all worth it if your oncologist pops into your exam room with a smile on his face and says, "Jim, there is no evidence of disease!"

Those are the words my doctor told me today! My scans came back clear showing no sign of cancer!!! Amen!!! Hallelujah!!! We have been rejoicing in our house this morning! What a huge relief to know that we can start putting life back together again without the threat of more chemo treatments.

As we drove up to Paradise this morning to meet with my oncologist, Dr. Mazj, I was beyond anxious. I couldn't focus on anything. My heartbeat was speed-metal fast. Waiting for test results pulls so many triggers for me, reminding me of getting the news I had cancer, reminding me that I had to have surgery, that I had to have chemo, that I wasn't done with chemo after round eight, reminding me that I'm fighting for my life. I was hoping for the best, but preparing for the worst all morning long. Fortunately, we received the best news possible. No more cancer! My liver is returning to normal, my blood counts were normal, and my body is stabilizing. Yes!

It seems surreal because I've lived with cancer and chemo and bad news for so many months. NED, this amazing news, hasn't found a home with me, though I am thrilled beyond belief that I received it. The possibilities seem to be piling up. No chemo? Sweet! But what does that mean? What will I do with all that time I spent fighting cancer, getting chemo, and waiting? What can I do now? I imagine it is like a person who retires and now has a plethora of time on his or her hands. How will I fill my days? The world seems wide open and full of possibilities. It is strange yet wonderful! God is so good and faithful.

From the doctor's office we drove straight to the kids' school, pulled them out of class and told them the good news right there on the playground with tears in our eyes. All we could do was grab each other and have a "whole family" hug. What a scene we must have been! But hey, when you are told you are NED, convention and self-awareness fly out the window and you cry, hug, and celebrate! Emily and I have been calling and texting everyone we can think of to share the good news. We can't seem to call and text enough. What a great problem to have!

I'll get my port removed from my chest next week, too. I'm so ready to have it out so I can wrestle with my kids again without pain. I will also be able to really start exercising without the disruption it causes.

Before taking the drive up to the hospital and receiving the news of NED, I reminded myself that if I got the news that I still had cancer it wouldn't change who I am. I would still be the same guy who would have to face more challenges. I guess in some ways receiving good news that I'm cancer-free is the same. I'm still the same old Jim. It's just that today I received really amazing news. It's so tempting to let my good circumstances (or bad) determine my identity. Today is just a great stitch in the larger tapestry of my life. I'll always treasure this day as the day that I was deemed "clear of all traces of cancer," and thank God for it, but I also want to put it into context with the bigger picture.

Not everyone gets to have a day like mine today, and for that, I am truly sad. I wish everyone got to experience what I'm experiencing because it's amazing. Our great comfort is that someday all will be made right and we will all get to celebrate our complete health and wholeness in the presence of God for eternity. Today is but a glimpse of that day, a foretaste, and a promise. If that day is anything like today, then I can't wait!

62 The Myth of Flatter Roads

November 16, 2009

The last few weeks have been a continuous celebration as we have raised many a glass in thanksgiving for the new life we've been given, a life set-free of cancer. Getting through the last year feels like the accomplishment of a lifetime. We have done battle with the evil forces of disease, disappointment, disillusionment, and depression. We have walked through the desert of our souls, been tried and tested in most every way. The strength of our wills, our bodies, and our family and friendship bonds have been put on trial, and the verdict was that we won! We are set free, even if just for a brief moment, from the chains of cancer.

Even as I count my lucky stars because I am well on the road to recovery, I am keenly aware that there will be more mountains to climb. I was on a walk with my mom last week and we were saying that we're ready for "normal" stress in our family—like deciding on what food to eat, whether or not my daughters should pierce their ears, and what shirt to wear in the morning. That would be nice. Our family has had a hell of time the past five or six years: Both sets of my grandparents have died, my dad was diagnosed with cancer and did chemo, several friends and family members have had miscarriages, and we've walked with many others through dark, trying times. Then I got cancer, had a major surgery, and did chemo for nine months. I'm ready for some flatter roads. I'm tired of the mountain climbs.

Once upon a time, during seminary, I used to ride my mountain bike in the Angels Crest National Forest outside of Pasadena. I remember, as I pedaled and pedaled and pedaled, hoping that the trail would flatten out and give me a rest from the continual climbing. But it seemed like it never did. I always felt that I was going up. It burned my lungs, and made my legs feel like stumps, barely able to crank another turn of the sprocket. Even now on my road bike I buy into the myth of flatter roads. As I round an uphill corner I imagine a nice flat section where I will be able to catch my breath, but again, the flatter roads don't usually appear; there seems to be just a lot of climbing.

So I made it through the uphill climb called colon cancer: Awesome! I'm so glad it's behind me; so glad we get to move on with the rest of the ride. But dang it! I can see more mountains ahead. I don't mean to sound cynical, but I need to keep my feet planted on earth and not allow myself to become a victim of the myth of flatter roads. Life is a series of climbs, of stresses, of problems to be solved, of obstacles, and issues: That's just the way life is. Sometimes we build our own mountains as we make silly, bad, or uninformed rash decisions. Yet other times the mountains just appear around the next blind corner, like being diagnosed with cancer when you are thirty-eight years old. I didn't see that mountain coming, but I had to climb none-the-less. After all, it wasn't your mountain, or my next-door neighbor's mountain…it was *mine*, all *mine* to climb.

If I've learned anything from cycling, and now cancer, it's that we have to keep climbing. We have to continue pedaling, keep turning over those gears one stroke at a time. To do any less is to deny the life we have been given and give up and turn our bikes around in defeat. That's lame. It's weak. It's rejecting the life God has given us.

It's not to say that we can't or shouldn't hop off and take some rests, eat some energy bars and take a long drink because we can't climb all the time—we should. Every now and then we need to stop and enjoy the view, take stock of how far we've come, and get geared-up for the remainder of the road ahead. It's also good to remember that not every mountain is an Everest.

But we can't buy into the myth of flatter roads, the myth that once we're done with a hard hill God or the universe somehow owes us the flats. It simply isn't true. We don't earn the rest we receive just like we aren't punished with the hills we are required to climb. To be sure, receiving times of rest is a wonderful gift. But if I've learned anything, it is that just around the corner another hill awaits us. It is all part of the journey and life we have been given. And we have to be determined to keep going, keep pedaling, because to do anything less is to stop living.

63 The Power of an Army

November 18, 2009

You have power. Did you know that? You have the power to change the world. Throughout the scriptures it seems that God listens to the prayers of his people. Like when a group of friends dug a hole in the roof of the crowded house and lowered their paralyzed buddy in front of Jesus in the hope that he might get healed in Luke 5. What did Jesus do?

> When Jesus saw their faith, he said, "Friend, your sins are forgiven."
> (Luke 5:20)

Jesus healed the man when he saw *the faith of his friends*. Wow! Somehow God uses the faith and prayers of friends to bring about healing and wholeness, God's *shalom*, to the world. That seems incredible!

God listens to the prayers of the few on behalf of the world. That's why he calls you the "salt of the earth" (Matt. 5:13). You're not the whole meal, but the salt on it. You give flavor and you preserve. You, my *Army of Love*, are the powerful, flavorful, preserving salt of the earth.

I remember many days when I couldn't even lift my head off the pillow to pray. But you could and you did, and God listened. I'm NED because, in large part, you prayed for it. You lowered me in front of Jesus and preserved my life. What a gift you have given me! God has heard your prayers and answered them!

As I walked Zoe this morning after last night's cool, refreshing rain, I was amazed at the beauty: Birds were singing, squirrels were dancing; today is a song. I have new life coursing through my veins because God has renewed and healed me. I appreciate days like today because I've had days full of crap where I wanted to die. But not so today. I'm alive today because God heard your prayers.

Thanks for praying and giving me new life. Keep after it. God listens to you. You can change the world. You changed me!

64 Coming Up On A Year

December 3, 2009

It was this time a year ago that I was in complete pain. My gut felt like it was run through with a sword throughout the Thanksgiving and the Christmas seasons. It was on Christmas day when all hell broke loose and the horror of cancer set in. So as we put up our Christmas tree and decorated our home tonight with carols playing in the background, I couldn't help but sense the dark cloud of last year looming close by, lurking at our windows like a burglar casing the joint. The carols, the ornaments, the smell of fresh-cut pine and spiced cider all remind me of the stench of cancer. That must be how anniversaries of this type are: Painful reminders of the hell and horror we've lived through. Will Christmas ever be sweet and joy-filled again? I hope so.

My little Advent reading this morning reminded that Jesus, who is the Light, came into the darkness, and the darkness did not understand the Light (John 1). The challenge, as I understand it, is to allow the Light to come into the darkness of this anniversary and drive out the shadows and fear. It is to let the purity, power, and truth of God's life and love replace the darkness and cold that cancer left behind.

It is a tall order to allow the light of Christ to drive out the darkness because, as much as I hate the darkness, I'm used to it. I've felt my way around in the dark. It has become my companion, my comfort, and my friend. It is where much of this year has been lived, so I'm not entirely sure what it means to live in the Light. Does it mean to forget? I can't: The scars won't let me. Does it mean to drive cancer and chemotherapy far from my mind? I can't: The pain was too searing, too deep to forget. Does it mean to not talk about it? How can I? Cancer is part of my story now. It has etched its scars into who I will be for the rest of my life. So how do I now live in God's light knowing the darkness so intimately? I don't know. I guess that's the wonder of Christmas:

> And the light shineth in darkness; and the darkness comprehended it not.
>
> (John 1:5, KJV)

I am open to the light, but I'm just not sure I comprehend it on this strange, yet vivid anniversary.

> *God, let your light shine brightly on this,*
> *the darkest of seasons;*
> *Where faith meets misery,*
> *where light meets darkness,*
> *Where life meets death face to face.*
> *And you win.*
> *You always win in the end.*
> *Help us remember the end of the story*
> *as we step into the light-dark world we call home.*
> *Not always dark;*
> *shocked by your sudden and bright light;*
> *overwhelmed by your radiant glory birthed in flesh,*
> *bearer of home,*

King of Glory,
Lord of Lords.
Come Lord Jesus, Come
Light of life.
Amen.

65 New Beginnings

December 29, 2009

I found myself getting more and more anxious as the one-year anniversary of my diagnosis approaches. It was on Christmas day a year ago that I found myself on my toilet during Christmas dinner, emptying myself of what can only be described as bloody, nasty, tumor-soaked crap. As the day approached I slowly began to realize that God was redeeming this holiday. It didn't have to be a nightmare again; it is a new year. I don't have the tumor. I feel relatively normal. I don't have cancer.

There I found myself again on the same toilet on Christmas day a year later thinking, "We really need to do something about this room. This tiny room of horrors hasn't changed since a year ago, but everything else has. We need to do something about this bathroom!"

Early the morning after Christmas, it was quickly and rashly decided that we were going to remodel that little room of nightmares we called our master bathroom. After a few quick phone calls to line-up some qualified help, my brother-in-law and I dug into the room with pure adrenaline and some bloody-knuckles. By early evening the entire bathroom was sitting in my driveway in a giant pile.

It was truly cathartic tearing out the very space where I suffered the worst scare of my life. It was like surgically removing my tumor all over again, though with a little less precision and a lot more muscle. I didn't realize the nightmare that was trapped in that toilet. When we tossed the toilet into the dump trailer and it cracked in half, I felt that a new beginning was initiated. Good-bye 2009 and the hell it brought! Good-bye bathroom and the horrors it contained in my memories! Good-bye cancer and the threat it posed to my family, my soul, my mind, and my faith. Hello new beginnings!

66 Keep Livin'

January 25, 2010

Unpredictable. Ever-changing. Precarious. Life. The people I love are hitting some rough waters, some dark nights, some desert times. Cancers have returned and beaten them. Their final hours of life are now upon them. As I took in their hard, sad news today, I felt myself sink with their sadness. I've always been a deep feeler. (I would cry when *other kids* got in trouble when I was in grade school.) I cried tears today for my dear friends. As I did, I was faced with that same familiar choice: Let the circumstance define me or define the circumstance; get tossed about by the waves or surf them; get blown away by the winds or fly a kite.

I drew another line in the sand.

The words, "keep on livin'" rang in my ears. Keep on livin'—circumstances are just that: circumstances. They don't have the power to rule us. They don't have the right to take over our minds, hearts, and souls—unless we give them that right. Cancer would have us believe that it is a death sentence. *Screw that.* It isn't a death sentence. It may be able to kill the physical, but it can't touch the spiritual hidden parts of our lives. Those parts are "hidden with Christ in God." (Col. 3:3) Those parts remain alive because God is alive.

I found myself defying cancer yet again as I drove through huge rain puddles, listened to country music really loud, and poured out my heart and angst to God. I worked hard and sweat it up at the gym, drank a latte, and made myself available for the adventure of loving others today. I am determined to keep on living even though death and sorrow knock at the door. I know they're out there. I'm just not inviting them in today.

67 Anniversaries Suck

February 3, 2010

I always thought that anniversaries were good things. Emily and I have been married for almost eighteen years and we've had some good celebrations of our marriage. There was the time we renewed our vows at a winery in Sonoma. Or the time I gave her a ruby ring at a little Italian restaurant. Then there was the time we celebrated on the shores of Maui. Those were good anniversaries.

But this one sucks. It is an anxiety-producing, sleep-losing, jaw-clenching, memory-inducing, fingernail-biting, back-tightening, stomach-aching anniversary from hell. I don't want to remember this date, that series of events, those tests, that surgery, and especially that freakin' chemo. Remembering those things brings back frailty. It brings back fears. It brings back stress. I am reminded that I have a chink in my armor, a dent in my fender, a pothole in my road. Cancer anniversaries suck.

I have successfully moved forward since the end of chemo. I've returned to work. I've returned to the gym. I'm back on the bike. I get to eat what I want. I'm not a slave to my bed. There are even whole hours when I don't think about cancer! Wow! But this one-year anniversary of my diagnosis has shackled me all over again.

I really have no solid evidence for my concern: My blood-work was great at my three-month check up last week, and tomorrow I go in for my one-year colonoscopy. I don't anticipate any bad news. But the mere fact of having to do it, to go back to the same place where I was told I have cancer a year ago is like returning to Ground Zero—just not a place I want to return to.

I look forward to telling everyone that I have the "all-clear" in a day, but until then, I covet prayers. I am reminded that this is a battle for my mind. I long to make today about God and his work through me, not about anniversaries, colons, bowel preps, tests, fasting, and fear. Pray that I stay in God's light where the darkness of anniversaries cannot touch.

68 It Starts With The Shoes

February 11, 2010

Yesterday I was at the gym trying to get my body back in some sort of shape. As I was suffering on the stationary spinning bike, an older gentleman of about seventy walked by. It was clear that he and the gym hadn't met in several years. His belly poured over his worn-out sweat pants, eyes darting back and forth wondering where he should start. Lift weights? Stationary bike? Stair climber? Zumba? Treadmill? He shuffled around for a few minutes before he disappeared to the back of the gym, but I could immediately tell he was committed to doing something: *It was in his shoes.*

His shoes were brand-new, top of the line Nikes. Just out of the box, not a scuff or speck of dirt anywhere on them—they were some sweet kicks. They were some serious athletic shoes begging to be worn by a determined, would-be athlete. This guy was going to get in killer shape. It was all in his shoes.

It all starts with the shoes. Sometimes—in fact, most of the time—it takes an act of sheer will to get through some of life's toughest spots like cancer. It may start with getting up off the couch, or making a phone call, or asking for help. It might be a simple prayer to God…or buying a new pair of shoes.

We have to start somewhere, but when we do we are defying our circumstances, drawing a line in the sand, and moving forward. Too often we allow the size of our circumstances get in the way of doing something. Consider Haiti in the wake of the recent devastating earthquake. We see their need and we tend to think, "What can one person do? What difference can I make?"

Strap on the new shoes and start walking. It may be a small step, but it is a step. It gets momentum going. It builds a head of steam. When we hear the words, "You have cancer," and you think, "I can't win this battle," make a phone call. Say a prayer. Show up and live. Don't let it defeat you before you even make an effort. Lace up those Nikes! Nothing has the right to steal our lives except that which we allow to become our burglar.

I am thankful for that seventy-year old pot-bellied athlete. He and his shiny Nikes reminded me that I need to keep pedaling and remain determined to live. That's what I'm going to keep doing, one day at a time, one moment at a time—starting right now.

Notes

Chapter 1: Christmas 2008

[1] Berry, Dave. "A Journey Into My Colon—and Yours." *Miami Harold*, February 22, 2008.

Chapter 3: The Truest Thing

[1] Lewis, C.S. *The Lion, The Witch, and the Wardrobe* (Scholastic, 1950), 163.

Chapter 26: I Like It!

[1] Matthews, Teresa K. *Cancer: The Adventure of Your Life!* (Teresa K. Matthews, 2001), 11.

Chapter 27: Taking The Risk

[1] Burchett, Andrew. "Place at the Table" on the CD, *Proof In The Mirror* (Andrew Burchett, 2005).

[2] Lewis, C.S. *The Problem of Pain* in *The Complete C.S. Lewis Signature Classics*, (Harper One, 2002), 604.

Chapter 49: Obstacles into Opportunities

[1] Armstrong, Lance with Jenkins, Sally. *It's Not About the Bike: My Journey Back to Life* (Berkeley Books, 2001), 37.

[2] Although Lance Armstrong has been stripped of all his awards due to the drug charges and findings, my respect for him as a cancer survivor remains high. His example of how to fight this disease has been life giving for my family and me. His professional and personal mistakes do not change my admiration of this man.

Made in the USA
San Bernardino, CA
04 May 2013